CANDLELIGHT BOOKS

Heroes and Villains
The *COVID-19*
Book of Lists

Reid Sheftall, M.D. received a physics degree from M.I.T. in 1978 and became a member of the University of Southern California faculty at age21. After a two-year stint as a card counter in Reno and Las Vegas, he moved on to medical school, surgery residency and a fellowship in Pediatric Burn Reconstruction. While completing his training in plastic and reconstructive surgery, Dr. Sheftall founded the charity Operation Kids to provide free surgery for burned and disfigured children of the developing world. After 28 years in private practice, Dr. Sheftall returned to training; this time in pediatric cardiac surgery.

During his time in Southeast Asia, Dr. Sheftall earned his tour card on various professional golf tours in Asia and played for 15 years, winning twice. Due to accumulating injuries, he decided to retire from professional golf at age 63. He played his final event as a member of the Asian Development Tour in 2019.

During the last two plus years, he has written hundreds of essays and made dozens of videos in an attempt to help the public understand SARS-2, COVID-19 and various treatments including the mRNA vaccines.

Dr. Sheftall is also the author of "The NO WILLPOWER DIET: *How to Slim Down To Your Ideal Weight Without Ever Being Hungry*". He wrote it in early 2020 in an attempt to assist people in losing the weight they needed to lose to reduce their chances of a bad outcome if they were to become infected with the SARS-2 virus. Dr. Sheftall created an approach to losing weight that does not involve counting calories or denial. It has been universally-successful with zero recidivism in two-and-a-half years. Fifteen years prior to that, he wrote "STRIKING IT RICH: *Golf in the Kingdom with Generals, Patients and Pros*", a memoir covering the first year of his return to golf at age 47 after a 30 year hiatus from the game. The book chronicles his attempt to gain a professional tour card within 12 months by going from local tournaments, to high stakes gambling games with the highest ranks of the Cambodian military, to Monday qualifying on the Thai Singha Tour, and finally to the Asian Tour Qualifying School at the end of the year. Dr. Sheftall divides his time between Phnom Penh, Cambodia and Ho Chi Minh City, Vietnam.

Heroes and Villains

The COVID-19
Book of Lists

Reid Sheftall M.D.

Contributions by Michael Yeadon PhD

CANDLELIGHT BOOKS

Candlelight Books, U.S.A.
#10 S. 3rd Street
San Jose, CA 95113

German, French, Japanese, Korean, Chinese, and Vietnamese translations are available. For information regarding special discounts for bulk purchases, contact Candlelight Books/Special Sales at the address above.

Manufactured in The United States of America

ISBN: 9798359969406 (Soft cover)

Also by Reid Sheftall, M.D.

THE NO WILLPOWER DIET: How to Slim Down to Your Ideal Weight, Without Ever Being Hungry
STRIKING IT RICH: *Golf in the Kingdom with Generals, Patients, and Pros*
THE TOURPLAYER'S HANDBOOK: Strategic Decisions, *Under Pressure,* in Tournament Golf
PHYSICS AND THE GOLF OF MATH MEDICINE

Coming soon…

IF ONLY THEY HAD LISTENED: *How I Cracked the Biggest Crime in Medical History*

To Henry Phan

Henry is the son of Tina Phan, my business partner and friend for 30 years. Before 2022, Henry was a delightful young man in his 30s. He graduated from Law school like his older sister Mai, but chose to work in the family business of hotel construction and management. Henry was a whiz with computers. He was in charge of advertising and reservations in addition to managing the newest and largest property in the portfolio.

In late March of 2021, Henry received his first dose of the Pfizer BioNTech vaccine. He received his second dose three weeks later in accordance with protocol. Six months after that, in September of 2021, Henry received his booster dose as recommended by the CDC.

Approximately two weeks after his booster dose, Henry began to feel numbness in his right arm, dizziness, and loss of balance. He was taken to the emergency room where radiological tests revealed a saddle thrombus at the bifurcation of his left common carotid artery and 90% occlusion of his left anterior descending, circumflex and right coronary arteries.

Virtually all of his coronary system was in need of bypass. He recovered from the transient ischemic attack and returned home with follow-up scheduled for peripheral vascular and cardiovascular surgery within the week. Henry was given general instructions to slim down- he was only moderately overweight, not obese- and to switch to a heart-healthy diet. When Henry was in ideal physical condition, he would undergo cardiac bypass surgery. Henry and I discussed his choice of cardiac surgeon many times as I had just completed training in that specialty. I was there every day supporting his effort to maximize his physical health in preparation for surgery.

Henry accepted his new challenge like nothing I have ever seen. He completely changed his diet and exercised daily. Henry didn't have 30 pounds to lose, but he lost them anyway, lowering his weight from 168 lbs to 134 lbs over the course of three months. His labs were spectacular. I've never seen such low cholesterol and triglycerides. Henry drove me to the airport for a three month trip overseas. I knew he would be having his surgery while I was gone.

On March 3, 2022, Henry received five bypasses to his coronary arteries.

The operation proceeded without incident and Henry was taken to the coronary care unit in stable condition, breathing on his own, and responding to verbal stimuli. After sleeping through the afternoon Henry was visited by his uncle David and fiancé, Thuy. He was able to converse easily.

The next morning, Henry's cardiac surgeon was unable to get him to respond. He had had a stroke in his left middle cerebral artery during the night. He could not move his right side or speak. He stayed in the ICU for six weeks.

Henry had been in rehab for over a month when I returned from overseas and saw him for the first time at his cardiac surgeon's office. Henry was full of emotions and wept freely when he saw me; more so when I bent over to hug him in his wheelchair.

I had known Henry since he was a small boy; before he was even old enough for school. His parents and older sister lived nearby and treated me like a member of their family, frequently inviting me over for dinner. They knew I was single, helpless, fairly hopeless, and worked very long hours as a surgeon just starting out. I tried to return what they had so generously given to me by helping everyone in their extended family with medical issues but it paled in comparison. The first memory I have of Henry was of him refusing to eat anything that wasn't colored white.

When I was in California on my way back to Florida, I worked regularly with Henry on his speech, and writing. I'm not sure if he improved in a month of helping him enunciate his words and write the letters of the alphabet. We had to teach Henry from first and second grade books. The strokes had affected his cognitive abilities very significantly. This was the hardest thing for me to see, given Henry's exceptional intellect prior to surgery.

Throughout the month that I worked with Henry, I never understood whether or not he knew what had happened to him. Then one day when we were writing letters, he scribbled something that no one else in the world would have been able to read, even his mother. In all the scribbles, I could pick out two words: "what happened?"

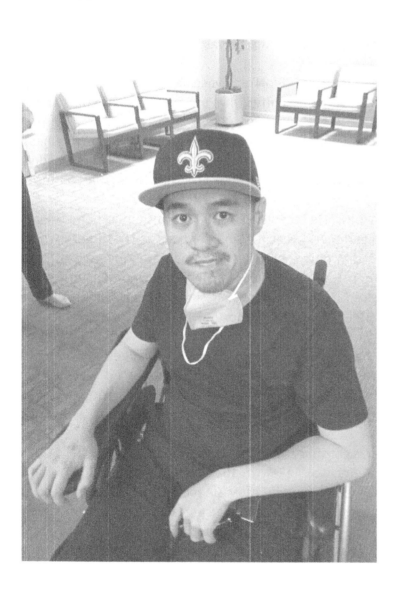

Table of Contents

Preface

I'm going to cut to the chase.

This is not going to end until we start naming names and filing charges. What we went through the last two plus years isn't the first time this has happened.

In January of 1976, a substantial number of soldiers stationed at Fort Dix, New Jersey, complained of a respiratory illness. Samples were sent to the N.J. public lab that serviced Fort Dix. It hit one of the soldiers, Private David Lewis, particularly hard. He was still sick in bed five days later when his company participated in a five-mile, forced march. Private Lewis got out of bed to join his fellow soldiers. During the march, he collapsed. His sergeant applied mouth-to-mouth resuscitation and Private Lewis survived, only to die a few days later. The sergeant never became ill.

The New Jersey lab identified most of the samples as the ordinary strain of flu going around that year but they were not able to identify the strain in four of the soldiers and in Private Lewis. The samples were sent to the CDC in Atlanta. A few days later, the CDC lab identified the samples as being a strain of Swine influenza A H1N1. By this time the other four soldiers had recovered without incident from the supposed swine influenza. Note that they recovered fully *without* a vaccine.

In February, CDC Director Dr. David Sencer distributed a memo calling for mass immunization for the swine flu. A month after that, President Ford was officially notified of the outbreak and endorsed the idea of mass immunization.

The vaccine manufacturers made two demands: 1) that there must be a guaranteed profit for the manufacturers, and, 2) that the government provide the manufacturers with indemnity from liability for any adverse effects arising out of the, as yet to be manufactured, vaccine. Both demands were met and the vaccination was manufactured and run through a testing protocol.

But something odd happened. The vaccines that got administered were not the ones tested. They used a different vaccine that was developed later but never tested in the kind of trials we have come to expect when new injections are introduced to the public.

The administration of the untested vaccine began on October 1, 1976. A year later, when asked if the vaccines were tested before being administered to the general public, Dr. Sencer said, "I…can't say. I would have to… I don't know. I would have to check the records. I haven't looked at this for some time."

What!? He was the Director of the CDC. He formulated the plan and was in charge of the vaccine rollout. It was his "baby". How could he not know they hadn't tested the vaccine?

But there was an even bigger problem. It turns out, over the nine months that elapsed between the Fort Dix outbreak- at this point looking very questionable- and the date of first injection, there was never a single additional case of swine flu confirmed anywhere in the world. "There had been several cases reported by the news media, but none confirmed", admitted Dr. Sencer.

Nine months is a very long time for not a single case of the disease popping up somewhere. Dr. Sabin, the inventor of one of the polio vaccines, wrote an editorial in the New York Times entitled "Washington and the Flu" in which he argued for a "wait-and-see" strategy by stockpiling the vaccines until it was clear they were needed. His advice was ignored.

In just the first month, three recipients died from heart attacks shortly after being vaccinated at the same Pittsburg clinic. That batch was recalled but vaccination continued. More and more recipients contracted Guillain-Barre Syndrome (GBS), a nervous system disorder that can cause paralysis and death.

The vaccine rollout continued through the Fall and early Winter months. During all this time, not a single additional case of Swine Flu was found. The GBS cases, however, were accumulating rapidly. The vaccines were finally discontinued on December 15, 1976, after 45 million people received the injection. 362 recipients across America contracted Guillain-Barre Syndrome and many died or were left paralyzed. The survivors (or the families of the deceased) applied for compensation from the U.S. Government since the manufacturers were granted indemnity from liability.

The case of the Swine Flu "outbreak" and vaccine launch of 1976 is not the same as the COVID-19 pandemic and vaccine launch of 2020, but there are some similarities and a few important lessons to take home. Similarities include, 1) the lack of informed consent provided to the recipients, 2) pharmaceutical industry shenanigans such as switching to a formulation that was not tested properly, 3) the incompetence, fraud, and prevarication that came out of the CDC and the attempts of the Director to cover up what was done, 4) the U.S. government's aggressive advertising campaign to get people to take the vaccines and 5) the President's participation at the time, urging people to get vaccinated without any justification for it.

There was no justification for pressuring the public to get these vaccines. In the case of the Swine Flu in 1976, nobody actually had the disease and in the case of COVID-19, we knew that the vaccine did not perform as promised. The real world vaccine data never came close to meeting safety and efficacy standards given that the original disease had an infection fatality rate of .1% for all ages and much lower than that in those under 60. The risk was tiny in young adults and negligible in children, reaching a risk of death of only one-in-a-million in small children. Nevertheless, the vaccines were approved and continue to be pushed to this day by government doctors such as Ashish Jha and CDC Director Rochelle Walensky for children as young as six months of age. The trials did not justify approval in this age group, let alone a campaign to promote them to new mothers.

The 1976 consent form everyone was asked to sign did not disclose the risk of potential side effects such as Guillain-Barre Syndrome. The forms only mentioned sore arm, fever, muscle aches, etc. This is exactly what happened with the Covid-19 vaccines. Parents were not warned about complications such as myocarditis, by the people administering the jabs even after the CDC knew about the increased risk.

In 1977, Dr. Sencer claimed he was not told GBS and other neurological complications were part of the risk profile. A younger member of the team, however, stated that he absolutely had informed Dr. Sencer and others regarding potential neurological complications including GBS, before the rollout commenced. How did he know? He did a search of the literature.

The take home lesson from all of this is that because we never punished the perpetrators for their egregious acts in1976 and several similar examples of the same thing since then, we had to live through it again this time.

It is my belief that if we had prosecuted the people responsible for the 1976 debacle, and sent them to prison if found guilty, almost fifty years of public abuse at the hands of Big Pharma would have been averted or greatly reduced.

And it's not just Big Pharma. Much of the abuse is carried out by their minions: the FDA, CDC, NIH, NIAID, mainstream media, social media companies and woke doctors everywhere. They are all in the pocket of Big Pharma as are the medical journals, credentialing agencies including certification Boards and just about any other medical association you can think of including the AMA and the various specialty associations. If they don't tow the party line- in this case the narrative leading to billions of vaccines sold, their funding will get cut off. This applies to politicians as well. If they upset the apple cart by telling the truth, Big Pharma's enormous contributions to their re-election campaigns will dry up overnight.

I've heard it said by many that we should not assign blame for what went on, that we should only want to find out what happened so we don't repeat the same mistakes during the next pandemic.
I say: No! Enough of this! People died and had their lives ruined because of what these people did. They do it every time a pandemic comes around and in the case of COVID-19, the death and destruction was orders of magnitude greater.

Aside from the loss of life and livelihoods of hundreds of millions of people, great suffering will occur secondary to the monetary indiscretions and out-and-out theft that occurred. People are already feeling it in the form of inflation through higher prices at the grocery store and elsewhere. In every case since 1976, the taxpayers have had to come in and pay for the damage done.

Did anyone commit prosecutable crimes this time around? Yes, they did.

The SARS-2 virus was constructed in a lab using taxpayer money while a moratorium was in place on gain of function research critical to that construction.

China kept the release secret for at least four months. They lied to the world with the help of the WHO, who proclaimed the virus unable to be transmitted from person to person. The truth is the virus was transmissible from person to person as soon as it was out of the lab. The designers made sure of that.

China then produced and released fake videos meant to scare Americans primarily, into accepting destructive policies like lockdowns, school closings, and mask mandates for the general public, It didn't hurt that Neil Ferguson and his group of modelers at Imperial College, London also pushed for these measures after publishing wildly inaccurate overestimations of the number expected to die followed by demands that those same non-pharmaceutical interventions- lockdowns and a few others-be adopted. Given Dr. Ferguson's track record, one has to wonder why, with a few notable exceptions such as Sweden, every country in the world agreed to his recommendations at almost precisely the same time.

Millions and millions of people had their livelihoods taken from them. According to a study commissioned by the WHO, supply chain disruptions secondary to the lockdowns are expected to cause over 100 million people to starve to death. The lockdowns did nothing beneficial such as slow the spread or flatten the curve despite what people were led to believe. And the people who understood why and wanted to share it with the world to prevent this disaster from happening, were censored by social media. Should the censors be punished for their contributions to the death and destruction? Of course they should.

What about the mainstream media show hosts who pushed the false Narrative? Should they be punished? Yes, they should.

Then came the vaccines pushed on the public with no justification. At certain points in time, they were mandated or set as a requirement to keep one's job. They were used to limit people's freedom to move about as they pleased even though they did not block transmission. Should pharmaceutical executives who manufactured the injections be prosecuted for malfeasance and collusion in choosing the spike protein when there were more effective and safer choices available? What about the government employees such as Drs. Fauci and Walensky and the media show hosts such as Rachel Maddow who lied about the vaccines' inability to block transmission for 5 months after this was known?

Never forget that people died and had their lives destroyed because of what these criminals did before they walked away with trillions of dollars. I'd like to see all of the people who engaged in the fraud be forced to return all of their ill-gotten gains a la the Bernie Madoff scandal. It would be very easy to do.

Publicly traded pharmaceutical companies made out like bandits. Moderna had never even brought a product to market before this outrageous scandal. They stayed alive through grants from the U.S.

government totaling $2.5 billion of taxpayer money. How often does the U.S. government come in and fund *your* failing enterprise so *you* can walk away with the profits?

Why don't we demand Pfizer, Moderna, Johnson and Johnson and Astra Zeneca sell some stock and pay the taxpayers back. There, I just found 20% of the money.

Hospitals and hospital systems can be made to return the perverse incentives they received for putting vulnerable patients on ventilators unnecessarily, causing large numbers of them to die. What about the fraud of calling deaths that had nothing to do with COVID-19, "COVID-19 deaths"? Anyone who died with a positive PCR test got called a COVID death regardless of the cause. They had the positive test result they needed because the PCR was run to 40 doubling cycles and above. Viable virus stops being able to grow out of samples at around 30 cycles, yet the PCR tests were run to 40 cycles or more in hopes of getting a positive result by amplifying a tiny fragment of the viral RNA into positivity. A cycle threshold of 42, say, constitutes an increase of 4000 times over a cycle threshold of 30. That led to many false positives which increased the case, hospitalization and death counts. The hospitals were happy to do it and the government was happy they did. That's why they gave them so much of *your* money for doing it. We'd like to have that money returned too.

There's another 20%.

It's frustrating, infuriating, and heartbreaking to find out how many people were involved in this fraud and theft of the public coffers.

Listing the names of the people who perpetrated these egregious acts is the first step toward making them return the money they obtained through fraudulent means. Then we must make them pay for their crimes in a way that will encourage anyone in the future to think twice about doing the same. This means being put on trial and sent to prison if found guilty. Remember, people died and were maimed for the rest of the only life they have because of what the perpetrators did.

This is not an angry approach to solving the problem. It's not about revenge. But it absolutely must be done. It's the only way we can make our society better.

That was my sole reason for writing this book.

Part I

Chapter 1 (People)

5 People Who Must be Brought In Immediately By Congress and Interviewed Under Oath Regarding Their Role in Creating the SARS-2 Virus

Dr. Collins was the NIH Director in 2014 when they awarded a five-year, taxpayer-funded grant to Eco-Health Alliance (EHA) to continue research in China while a moratorium on gain of function research was in effect in the U.S. EHA was the New York-based non-profit run by British national, Peter Daszak, PhD. They took part of the money and subcontracted the laboratory work to the Wuhan Institute of Virology, run by Zheng Shi Li, PhD.

Dr. Shi had been working with Dr. Ralph Baric for several years prior to this. He had sent her "humanized" mice she needed to perform experiments measuring a bat coronavirus's ability to infect human lung cells and cause SARS-like symptoms. Humanized mice are mice that have human, as opposed to mouse, ACE-2 receptors on the surface of their lung and other cells.

In 2018, Dr. Daszak submitted a grant proposal to DARPA, asking for $14 million to continue the project after the original NIH grant was scheduled to expire. DARPA refused to fund EHA on the grounds that the research was too dangerous. Anthony Fauci stepped in to supply the taxpayer-funding necessary to continue the research.

1. **Peter Daszak, PhD**
2. **Francis Collins, M.D., PhD**
3. **Anthony Fauci, M.D.**
4. **Zheng Shi Li, PhD**
5. **Ralph Baric, PhD**

16 Most Prolific Censors

1. Susan Wojcicki

This woman is the YouTube CEO. Since the beginning of the pandemic, she has been authorizing the removal of videos that explain the correct basic science behind COVID-19 while allowing videos that contain grossly incorrect information to remain on the platform- not just misleading, wrong. She has been depriving people of the knowledge they could use to save their lives and those of their loved ones.

The YouTube Official Misinformation policy is in Appendix I and I urge you to read it. They consider "misinformation" to be many things that are actually true.

YouTube will take down videos that contain:

Example #1:

"Content that encourages the use of home remedies"

Certainly, gargling with salt water or even tap water would be considered a "home remedy".

Reducing the viral load can be very helpful, regardless of how you accomplish it. Numerous studies in the medical literature have confirmed the reduction in oropharyngeal viral load that results from gargling with tap water and/or hypertonic saline. One such article located at

https://www.ncbi.nlm.nih.gov/pmc/articles/PMC7266767/ states "A randomized trial in Japan showed that throat gargling with tap water 3 times a day significantly reduced the incidence of upper respiratory tract infection (UTRI) by 36%. Another randomized trial in England, showed that nasal cavity irrigation and throat gargling with hypertonic saline during 48 h after symptom onset in patients with URTI significantly reduced the period of illness by 1.9 days, the use of medications by 36%, household contact transmission by 35%, and the viral load significantly.

The possible reasons for the effectiveness of throat gargling may be that the physical washing agent used in throat gargling causes shedding of the virus and infected cells or causes the chemical inactivation of the virus. "

YouTube is wrong to take down videos that encourage newly-infected patients to try a so-called "home remedy" based on the results of legitimate studies that show a very inexpensive method for reducing in-home transmission of the virus that causes COVID-19, given that a significant number of transmissions occur in the home.

Recall that ER doctors were sending people home from emergency rooms, telling them there was nothing they could treat them with and to come back when they had difficulty breathing.

Example #2:

"Content that claims Ivermectin and Hydroxychloroquine are safe to use in the prevention of COVID-19".

I'm going to show you that both of these medications are very safe.

It is truly absurd that a person, Ms. Wojcicki, who majored in humanities and went to business school and knows almost nothing about medical science, is making a decision based on her incorrect understanding of the safety profile of two medicines, the use of which might save the lives of millions of people infected with the SARS-2 coronavirus.

HCQ is used for Malaria prophylaxis and treatment due to its anti-helminthic properties. Only very safe drugs are used for prophylaxis because you haven't gotten the disease yet. They are used to prevent you from *getting* the disease. Would it make any sense to give you a preventative that caused more morbidity and mortality than the disease it was preventing?

And yet in the judgment of Ms. Wojcicki, with all her accumulated medical knowledge, claiming HCQ is safe to use for the prevention of COVID-19 is so egregious an error that it justifies taking down a video and, in some cases, an entire channel.

Further proof that HCQ is safe:

HCQ is used in treating two autoimmune diseases due to its anti-inflammatory properties; Systemic Lupus Erythematosus and Rheumatoid Arthritis. These are diseases that last for very long periods of time: 30 years, 40 years, 50 years, etc. HCQ must be taken daily to keep these conditions under control. The initial dose for RA is 400mg to 600mg daily. This is reduced to 200mg to 400mg daily for long term treatment. For SLE, a dose of 200mg to 400mg is used daily. The dose for COVID-19 prophylaxis is 200 mg-400 mg two times a week. Since HCQ is considered safe for use in RA and SLE where it is used at a much higher frequency for a much greater duration, it is unreasonable to think that these drugs are not safe for the prophylaxis of COVID-19. If this drug is effective in the prevention of COVID-19 as many clinical doctors claim, the actions of YouTube in not allowing videos to be shown that endorse the safety of HCQ in COVID-19 prophylaxis most definitely contribute to the deaths of some patients who would have learned about it from those videos and benefitted from its use.

Now, Ivermectin (IVM)

I won't belabor the point but, again, IVM is used as a prophylactic, in this case for River Blindness. You don't use medicines as prophylactics if they aren't safe. IVM is a very safe medicine.

Example 3:

"Content that recommends use of Ivermectin for the treatment of COVID-19"

Ms. Wojcicki is responsible for depriving the public of receiving recommendations to use an effective medicine used to treat a deadly disease.

Example 4:

"Categorical claims that Ivermectin is an effective treatment for COVID-19"

Ms. Wojcicki authorized the taking down of a video in which Dr. Bhattacharya and I presented the results of studies published in the literature; two well-meaning medical doctors discussing a topic of interest to the public about how to protect themselves from a deadly disease. No categorical claims were made, just statements along the lines of, "There's only one study here out of about 30 that doesn't show efficacy. This looks like it works to me." We were very conservative in our comments.

It's too bad for the people supporting the Narrative. When it comes to the efficacy of IVM in treating COVID-19 (for the proper cohort at the proper dose for the proper duration), the literature is overwhelmingly in favor of the claim, "Ivermectin is an effective treatment for COVID-19. Look at the results of this study; a meta-analysis of randomized, controlled trials: (please start watching at 4:30) https://www.youtube.com/watch?v=yOAh7GtvcOs&t=12s

Example 5:

"content that claims COVID-19 vaccines do not reduce risk of serious illness or death"

Wrong again. There is no question that considering death from all causes, the COVID-19 mRNA vaccines not only DO NOT reduce serious illness and death, they INCREASE serious illness and death. Numerous studies demonstrate this.

Example 5:

"content claiming that vaccines do not reduce transmission"

I proved the vaccines don't block transmission in mid- January of 2021C and told the world through videos I posted on YouTube. That was only one month after the vaccines had been released to the public. Many people would have wanted to know if the vaccines were incapable of blocking transmission. They may not have wanted to get the vaccines if they had known this. Even Drs. Fauci and Walensky have come around now, and admit the vaccines don't block transmission, yet YouTube is still taking down videos that "claim vaccines do not reduce transmission".

YouTube increased deaths in two ways by taking these videos down.

1. Many of the people who would not have gotten the vaccine if they had been allowed to see the videos, have died from vaccine-related side effects.

2.The false security of thinking the vaccines protected the recipient from getting infected, caused them to let down their guard and engage in riskier behavior, resulting in more of them getting infected and eventually dying.

2. Sundar Pichai, Alphabet C.E.O.

As it is Sundar Pichai's job to oversee Susan Wojcicki, everything that applies to her applies to him. Pichai has an engineering background and while it doesn't mean he knows anything about medical science, he should possess enough analytical skill to determine if a drug is safe or not and even if it is efficacious in treating a disease. He definitely played a role in censoring information that could have been used to save lives.

On top of all this, Wojcicki and Pichai left up videos that disseminated false information, thereby putting people at higher risk of getting and dying from COVID-19.

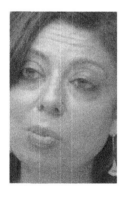

This is Monica Ghandi, M.D. She was on a podcast by Z-Dogg. He posts comedy and medical videos on YouTube. They left this video up for more than two years even though almost all of it is wrong and very dangerous. These two doctors believe that masks work, for example, and that's not even 5% of it. Here's the link: https://www.youtube.com/watch?v=N8N5oduX1KQ&t=2400s When the public watch something like this, they believe most of it because these two doctors are supposed to know something. They then engage in the behaviors endorsed here. Some of them will die because of it because they get a false sense of protection.

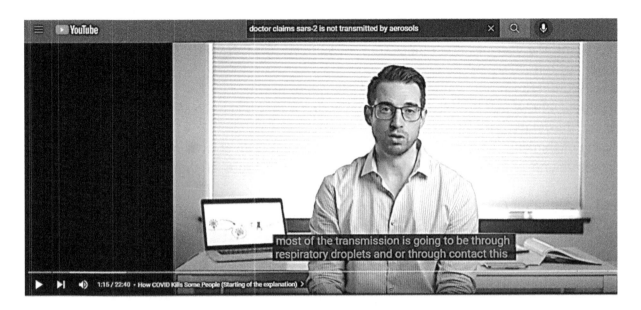

This is a screenshot of one such video, left up for two years and counting. It features a doctor claiming the virus is transmitted primarily by respiratory droplets (that fall to the ground quickly) and by contact. This is absolutely incorrect and very dangerous misinformation. The virus is transmitted by aerosols, primarily. Aerosols can stay in the air for hours or even days. The falsehood relayed by this doctor puts people at risk because they are misled as to how the virus is transmitted. They will miss the chance to modify their behavior and reduce their risk of becoming infected. This video is still up after more than two years having garnered more than 6.7 million views (of false information, remember) while some of my videos that contain no falsehoods or misleading statements, get taken down in minutes, sometimes with less than 10 views.

Take a look at this video: https://www.youtube.com/watch?v=fygh-0THA7k
Wojcicki and Pichai left it up. It's full of stupidity and false claims compliments of Senator Jack Reed of Rhode Island, CDC Director Robert Redfield, Admiral Brett Giroir, and Dr. Robert Kadlec.

Here is one from Chris Hayes's show on MSNBC: Mrs. Wojcicki has left this one up since it was posted on June 21, 2021. It is FULL of false and dangerous information that undoubtedly resulted in the deaths of some who watched this. https://www.youtube.com/watch?v=OrjMLONm-Bw

Here are a few other examples, compliments of Rachel Maddow. These are still up. Today is September 15, 2022.
https://www.youtube.com/watch?v=tj6EkqfCRbA
https://www.youtube.com/watch?v=6LQMvABRTLQ
In these videos, Rachel is urging people to get the vaccine, telling them, incorrectly, that if you are vaccinated, you can't get the virus and you can't spread it to anyone else. This is the exact opposite of reality and very, very dangerous. YouTube has left these videos up while having taken mine down because they contain my explanation that the vaccines do *not* keep a person from getting infected or from passing it on to someone else, which is actually true. Certainly, lots of people died because they took her advice. Lots of people have offered the excuse that she "is not a doctor, so how could she have known about this." Exactly. If she doesn't understand the disease, she shouldn't be giving advice to her 3 million viewers. Back then, I think she was on every night. Think of the number of people who have died and will

die because of her doing this. Look at YouTube and Susan Wojcicki's responsibility for these deaths. People are dying because of Rachel's advice and they leave her video up. I would have saved hundreds of thousands of lives and they took mine down, saying it contained false and misleading information.

Wojcicki and Pichai have controlled the public discourse on a subject they know very little about by taking down and leaving up videos. They are putting millions of people at increased risk of severe disease and death by doing this.

Taking down my videos and others like them also puts people at risk. I'm very careful not to make a mistake. 1. I don't want to hurt anyone. 2. I wouldn't want it on my conscience. 3. I don't want to damage my reputation by putting up a video with even a tiny mistake in it.

There is not a single person employed at YouTube, Google or Alphabet, including their subcontractors, who knows as much as I about SARS-2, COVID-19 and the vaccines. They might have a right to take down my and others' videos while leaving up incorrect and misleading ones. I do not know. But that's not the issue here. The issue is that they are contributing to the deaths of innocent people by doing so.

3. Mark Zuckerberg, Facebook C.E.O.

Zuckerberg is notorious for removing helpful information from the Facebook platform in the same way YouTube does. You would think that his wife, Pricilla Chan, who is a doctor, would intervene. She must know, for example, that the vaccines don't block transmission of the virus. Facebook also takes down private support groups discussing treatments for COVID-19 and side effects of the vaccines. Private support groups are set up to help people get through an illness. It's disgraceful. Dr. Chan?

4. Jack Dorsey, Twitter C.E.O.

Almost everyone who has been helpful in educating the public has been bumped off of Twitter, many permanently. Again, this causes people to die unnecessarily. Numbers 1,2,3, and 4 also collude with the U.S. government to take down information that goes against "the Narrative" (see below).

5. Parag Agrawal, Twitter C.E.O.

He took over from Jack Dorsey on November 29, 2021. Everyone was hoping he wouldn't be as bad as Dorsey when it comes to censorship, but the silencing of helpful voices continues. "Twitter, like other private companies, isn't bound by the First Amendment', Agrawal said. I don't know if that's true or not but he's missing the point. It's not whether Twitter has a right to remove tweets that are correct on the science of SARS-2, COVID and the vaccines while leaving up those that spread false information. It's that he is contributing to the death toll by doing so

6. Carol Crawford

She is the CDC's liaison with employees of Google, Facebook and Twitter to censor voices that don't adhere to the Narrative. Emails have been uncovered in which she directs social media companies to censor what they call misinformation. Since the Narrative has been proven wrong over and over again on every major call, she is depriving people from getting information they could use to save their lives

7. Nick Clegg, Meta (Facebook)

Read the email below. It appears the people involved got caught red-handed.

From: Nick Clegg ◄████████████████████►
Date: Friday, July 23, 2021 at 7:29 PM
To: Murthy, Vivek (HHS/OASH) ◄████████████████████►
Cc: Guy Rosen ████████fb.com>, Brian Rice ◄██████e@fb.com>, Waldo, Eric (HHS/OASH)
<████████@hhs.gov>
Subject: Message from Nick Clegg

Dear Vivek (if I may),

Thanks again for taking the time to meet earlier today. It was very helpful to take stock after the past week and hear directly from you and your team, and to establish our next steps.

We talked about the speed at which we are all having to iterate as the pandemic progresses. I wanted to make sure you saw the steps we took just this past week to adjust policies on what we are removing with respect to misinformation, as well as steps taken to further address the "disinfo dozen": we removed 17 additional Pages, Groups, and Instagram accounts tied to the disinfo dozen (so a total of 39 Profiles, Pages, Groups, and IG accounts deleted thus far, resulting in every member of the disinfo dozen having had at least one such entity removed). We are also continuing to make 4 other Pages and Profiles, which have not yet met their removal thresholds, more difficult to find on our platform. We also expanded the group of false claims that we remove, to keep up with recent trends of misinformation that we are seeing.

Did you catch that? Meta (Facebook) deleted 39 Profiles, Pages, Groups, and Instagram accounts in an effort to remove what they deem "misinformation". You now know from reading the above that what they deem misinformation is not always that. I have no doubt that some of the material posted on Facebook and the other platforms is incorrect and/or misleading. I roll my eyes when I see it too. But some of my videos and posts have been taken down when there is absolutely nothing in them that is incorrect. There was no justification to remove any of my videos or posts or the private group I formed, "Every Blade of Grass". As soon as we reached 500 members, "poof" it was gone.

The other slip-up from Nick Clegg's message to Vivek Murthy, the Surgeon-General of the United States, is when he admits to Facebook's practice of making Pages and Profiles "more difficult to find on our platforms". I always wondered why my Pages, Posts and Videos got so few views on Facebook and YouTube. I suspected "shadow banning" and once wrote a few dozen of my Facebook friends to see if they had gotten a specific post of mine. They all answered, "No." When they weren't taking my posts and videos down, they were making sure no one saw them. Thank you, Nick Clegg.

If YouTube had a list of people they shadow banned as a matter of course, I was on it. My videos on COVID-19 got from 500 – 2000 views which is very low, no matter how good they were. Several announced breakthroughs of major importance to Covid-19 and the lives of people everywhere. Videos containing these major breakthroughs such as my derivation of the correct infection fatality rate got very few views while I watched non-doctors fumble their way through an explanation of something very simple, making mistake after mistake, all the way to 400,000 views. Part of the problem is that the public didn't understand any of this so a particular chiropractor I recall, who did not know anything about the human response, basically fooled viewers into thinking he did and his videos got close to a million views. One of my friends who is an architect told me once he enjoyed watching that guy's videos. Unfortunately, there's been a lot of that going on over the last few years.

They even took down a derivation of the correct infection fatality rate I posted on March 8, 2020. China Medical had it at 4%, the CDC at 3.2%, and Italy Medical 7%, I derived it from the Diamond Princess cruise ship data to be .1%. I made a few minor assumptions but they were perfectly reasonable. Dr. Levitt did the same thing and got something very close to me. I think his was .2%. If I remember correctly, that one was gone in three days. My proof that the vaccines were unable to block transmission (January 15, 2021), and the one showing we reached herd immunity to the Wuhan strain on January 11, 2021, were taken down within less than an hour. These videos would have saved millions of lives because they would have convinced people first, not to agree to the lockdowns for a virus with an IFR the same as the flu and second, not to get the vaccine given that it didn't block transmission and therefore didn't help us reach herd immunity (which we reached without a single person being vaccinated).

Drs. Fauci, Reiner and others claimed in late September, 2020 that 90% of the U.S. population was vulnerable to becoming infected. They were way off but since it went with the narrative, no one checked it. I knew they weren't counting immunity-in-place, T-cell and B-cell memory like the kind you get after you have been exposed to a virus. Actual antibody molecules stay in your blood only about three months. They had forgotten that too, evidently. If that doesn't seem possible to you given your protection from disease, consider the following. If you are 50 years old and had your measles vaccine when you were very young, you wouldn't have the antibodies in your blood that you produced after receiving the injections, right?. They *don't* last forever. But you *do* have T and B-cell memory to the antigens you were exposed to back then. They are ready to attack measles virus if you were to encounter it again. Those memory cells will mobilize rapidly, making new antibodies which will participant in killing the intruder before it gets into your cells and starts making copies of itself.

But Fauci, Reiner, etc. drew the incorrect conclusion that if only 10% of the people tested had active antibodies to SARS-2 in their blood, then 90% of us were still vulnerable. I don't know why these doctors didn't know something this basic. Maybe they knew it but didn't want to admit the truth because it would have destroyed interest in getting the vaccines. I really don't know. If they *are* faking it, their performances are Oscar-worthy.

Part of the reason people took the vaccine was to help us- society as a whole- reach herd immunity. If those same people had seen a video I posted in late September showing the true number of exposed plus those with immunity-in-place, they would have realized we would be reaching herd immunity sometime during the winter season, which we did. But YouTube took my videos down. (I do have screenshots and they are located at #4 in "**8 *Most Important Slides of the Pandemic***"). The serological tests they ran, found only 10 % of the population had antibodies circulating in their blood. To someone not familiar with clonal expansion and memory, they might conclude 90% of the population was still vulnerable. It's hard to believe Fauci and Reiner would not know how the immune system worked. Maybe they forgot. A lot of clinicians decades out of medical school, where they struggled to understand it in the first place, have forgotten what they knew a few decades down the road. Dr. Haseltine has a PhD. He is not a medical doctor so, depending on his field, he might not have ever learned this. He should get a pass as long as he doesn't comment on it. But he did comment on it. Ho once said, "Herd immunity is the equivalent of mass murder".

The bottom line is, they were all completely wrong. There weren't 90% of the U.S. population vulnerable to infection. The true number was about 15%. I proved it the same day as their CNN comments. I predicted that day in late September that we would reach herd immunity sometime in the winter season. I was vindicated three-and-a-half months later, right in the middle of the winter season. We got the final 15% or so during the winter bump as predicted and the cases vs. time curve dropped straight down. The virus couldn't find anyone else to infect that didn't have an immune response at the ready to ward it off. Those holding the view that 90% were still vulnerable, had forgotten about expansion and memory (155 million), immunity-in-place (120 million), t-cells, and the fact that almost all antibodies last only 3 months. If someone was infected before July, they wouldn't have been counted in their surveys at the end of September. When they thought 10% of the U.S. population of 350 million or 35 million were protected, there were actually about 275 million protected.

9. Joe Biden

The Attorneys General of Missouri and Louisiana are suing President Biden and members of his administration (10, 11, 12, 13, and others) for allegedly colluding with social media to censor and suppress truthful speech related to mask efficacy and the laboratory origin of the SARS-2 virus. In early August, the judge on the case gave the go ahead for discovery. Early days here- we'll have to wait and see what becomes of this.

11. Jen Psaki, Former Press Secretary

12. Vivek Murthy, M.D., Surgeon General of the United States here, and see 8.

I was SHOCKED to learn what Dr. Vivek Murthy was involved in. I don't know him. I don't know anything about him. But that job comes with an enormous platform and a responsibility to the public on health matters. Colluding with social media companies to deprive the public of information they could use to save their lives and those of their loved ones is antithetical to the mission of the Surgeon General.

13. Nina Jankowicz

Ms. Jankowicz is the former Director of the Department of Homeland Security's short-lived Disinformation Governance Board. It was "paused" after only three weeks under criticism from all sides as un-American to be policing the speech of American citizens. Nina Jankowicz resigned under public outcry. She had once said, "We should view [Hunter Biden's laptop] as a Trump campaign product".

14. Andy Slavitt (Senior Advisor to the COVID-19 Response Coordinator)

 Mr. Slavitt went to Wharton and Harvard business school. His first job was as an investment banker. In 2003, he sold a company he started, called Health Allies, to the HMO, United Health Group. He became CEO of Optum/Insight and the group executive vice president for Optum, both subsidiaries of United Health.

Five years later, in February of 2008, Optum, then named Ingenix, was investigated by New York State Attorney General Andrew Cuomo due to "**a scheme by health insurers to defraud consumers by manipulating reimbursement rates**." Less than one year into the investigation, on January 13, 2009, Ingenix announced an agreement with the New York State attorney settling the probe into the independence of the health pricing database. United Health Group and Ingenix would pay $50 million. On January 15, 2009, only two days later, UnitedHealth Group announced a $350 million settlement of three class action lawsuits filed in federal court by the American Medical Association, UnitedHealth Group members, healthcare providers, and state medical societies for **not paying out-of-network benefits**. He's a businessman, an executive in an HMO, a completely superfluous layer of profit takers situated between doctors and their patients, adding significantly to the cost of medical care. I can tell you from experience that these places make a lot of their money by collecting premiums and denying coverage. They do this by refusing to approve medically-indicated procedures and by denying payments to doctors after the procedure has been performed.

This actually happened to me in my first job. I was the only surgeon in a small town in Mississippi. All of the hospital employees used me as their surgeon. I was a novice at filing insurance claims and they kept sending them back. This went on for a year. After a year went by, the insurance company said they didn't have to pay because the claims were now past the time limit for submitting. They dragged their feet in notifying me that I had to re-submit my claims, sometimes by as much as three or four months. When I wrote them a letter, asking for the reason why the payments hadn't arrived, I heard once again that there was something wrong with the form I had sent in. After a year of this back and forth, letters came that said, "Please refer to Ms "So and So" for remittance." I wasn't about to bill the people who scrubbed the floors so I could walk around in my white coat all day. I think it was about 10 cases I didn't get paid for.

Mr. Slavitt wouldn't have even a freshman level understanding of what would constitute false and misleading information as it pertains to a pandemic caused by a coronavirus transmitted by aerosols, nor would he understand how the human immune system works and why the vaccines were unable to block transmission. He certainly would not understand how the vaccines worked or even the risks associated with their use. This probably was of no concern to President Biden who assigned him to the role of "Senior Advisor to the COVID-19 Response Coordinator". It was probably more valuable to the Narrative that the companies he ran and helped run got into trouble with the New York State Attorney General after only five years of his tenure there. The last thing Biden wanted, was a very knowledgeable medical doctor who would be unwilling to remove any information from social media that could benefit patients.

Along with 15 and 16, Mr. Slavitt worked with social media to try to get them to take down posts containing "false and misleading information" on COVID-19. Mr. Slavitt, Mr. Flaherty, who double majored in TVR and politics at Ithaca College, (i.e. no medical knowledge), and lawyer Dana Remus (no medical knowledge) were working with social media companies who also did not have any medical knowledge. Their mission was to take down false and misleading information on COVID-19 without either group actually knowing what was false and misleading. People died because of this.

A little research into "fact checkers" revealed that these companies rarely had employees doing the fact checking who had a background in any science, let alone medicine, and in all the companies I checked, there was not a single medical doctor; not that being a doctor makes one immune to spreading false and misleading information, just listen to Drs. Jha, Fauci, Walensky, Collins, Birx, Wen, Reiner, M. Gandhi, Sanjay Gupta, etc. My posts, which contained no false and misleading information, were regularly taken down while I watched doctors like the one pictured above, Dr. Mike Hansen, get things wrong at times, dangerously misleading the public. For example, his claim that the virus is transmitted primarily through respiratory droplets makes people confident that they can shop a grocery aisle 20 minutes after someone has lingered there because respiratory droplets fall to the ground rapidly. But that person should not be confident at all. Aerosols linger for hours or even days in stagnant, indoor air.

Let's not kid ourselves, though. The false information these doctors have been spreading since January of 2020 has only partially been due to lack of knowledge and understanding. They've also been motivated by money, power, fame, and political ideology to varying degrees.

   15. **Rob Flaherty(Deputy Assistant to the President)**
   16. **Dana Remus (White House Lawyer)**

31 Physicians/Scientists Most Brave in Challenging The Narrative

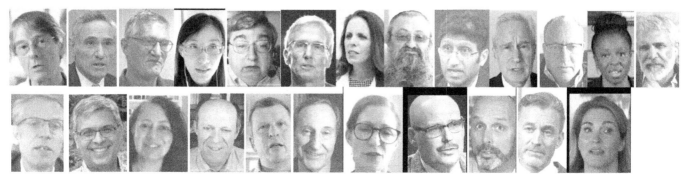

1. **Michael Yeadon, PhD**

   From the very beginning, Dr. Yeadon was incredibly insightful and brave in speaking out about all aspects of this major fraud. He provides the perfect example for all of us who might hesitate to speak up when we see an injustice. Some of us learn to stand up to injustice and bullying at age 10 in the schoolyard. Most learn later. We *all* have to have this skill as adults. Clearly, most members of the medical and lab research community have not learned this. They sat back and let this happen for 2 ½ years and counting. Not so, Dr. Mike Yeadon. He spoke up from day one.

   Very early on, Dr. Yeadon offered many insights regarding the grand plan someone had for the world; vaccine passports and so forth. He has been very brave in speaking out about the industry in which he worked for a few decades, even challenging his former colleagues by name. He was a VP at Pfizer before breaking off to form his own company, which he later sold.

2. **Scott Atlas, M.D.**

   Thank God for Dr. Atlas. He is a tough, no nonsense doctor who, as far as I can tell, was right about everything except for one tiny statement. I actually had him tied with Dr. Yeadon for the top spot until I found a video in which he said (paraphrasing) it was reasonable to try the lockdowns for a few weeks at the beginning because we didn't know at the time they wouldn't work. It's a tiny indiscretion, I know, but it's all I could find to separate him and Dr. Yeadon. I gave him a tiny demerit for that answer because I felt it *was* possible, before they were put into place, to know why lockdowns could not work and were actually the exact *opposite* of what should have been done.

   People know now that they were a dismal failure but not back then. Oh, the flak I received from family, friends, strangers and acquaintances over my proclamations regarding lockdowns in mid-March of 2020. I was sure I was right, though and wrote Tucker Carlson and Sean Hannity at FOX and Anderson Cooper and Chris Cuomo at CNN asking for five minutes of their time with which to explain "that we were heading for death and destruction on a biblical scale". None of them wrote back. I will tell the whole story with scientific detail in the book I am working on now, entitled, "If Only They Had Listened: *How I Cracked the Biggest Crime in Medical History*" with the word 'Medical' crossed out but you can still read it, implying that this was the biggest crime in history, not just medical history.. The release is about five months away. For now, (please see **"Most Important Slides of the Pandemic" in "Part I, Chapter III, Things"**)

   Dr. Atlas got attacked not only by know-nothings on the internet but by 106 of his former colleagues at Stanford University Medical Center. This is a book about naming names and holding people accountable so I listed each and every one of them. The first signer, which means it was he, who most likely wrote the letter, is a former Dean of the medical school, Philip A. Pizzo, M.D., a pediatrician. I shot the letter full of holes and called out Dr. Pizzo for not giving us examples of when Dr. Atlas "fostered falsehoods and misrepresentations of science." I hope he and the other 105 see this book and think about what they did.

   Dr. Atlas went on show after show without regard to political ideology as part of his job to help the public understand COVID-19 and the policies to combat it. Since most of the media are left-leaning, he had to endure shot after shot of invective. He kept his cool through it all.

   One memorable appearance was on Erin Burnett's CNN show. Like Rachel Maddow, she exposed her ignorance instantly and then told Dr. Atlas he wasn't qualified to work as an advisor in the White House because he was a radiologist in his earlier days Ever the gentleman, he calmly informed her, "For the last 10 years, I have worked and written on public health policy at the Hoover Institution at Stanford". She hadn't even reviewed her guest's background.

3. **Nils Anders Tegnell, M.D**

Sweden's State Epidemiologist. He got plenty of flak from his colleagues but resisted. Sweden provided the control group that saved the world. This man, and his Prime Minister, Stefan Lofgren deserve our eternal gratitude.

4. **Li-Meng Yan, M.D., PhD**

From an interview she gave over her first nine months here: Dr. Yan was working at the Hong Kong School of Public Health studying coronaviruses. Her boss was the WHO liaison for the region. He asked her to go to Wuhan on December 31, 2019 to find out what was going on and to report back to him. She was selected to go to Wuhan because she was the only one in her group who could speak Mandarin having attended school in mainland China.

She was warned not to cross the "Red Line" by the people in Wuhan or she would "get disappeared". "Crossing the red line" meant divulging what was being done there. She bravely went ahead and spilled the beans on China, telling the world on YouTube in Chinese that 1) China knew about the virus well before they told the world, 2) The virus could be transmitted from person to person, 3) SARS-2 mutated often, 4) The wet market was a "smokescreen" and, 5) the virus was made in a lab. She fled to the U.S. where she was granted asylum and lived in hiding in the early months. Dumb or corrupt officials in the U.S. told her she was wrong about the virus being created in the Wuhan Institute of Virology. We now know she was right.

Talk about brave, there are lots of Chinese agents in Hong Kong and the U.S. and every one of them would like to "get her disappeared". She has to be very careful. I hope she has good security.

5. **Richard Ebright, PhD**

The brilliant, Harvard-educated researcher **is** the Head of everything Molecular Bioscience at Rutgers University. He put his future funding at risk by telling the truth. Here is his assessment of the actions by the NIH and NIAID Directors: regarding their denials that gain of function research was conducted in Wuhan: "The NIH, specifically Collins, Fauci and Tabac lied to congress, lied to the press, lied to the public, knowingly, willfully, brazenly," and in response to Dr. Fauci's assertion that "the NIH and NIAID categorically have not funded gain of function research to be conducted in the Wuhan Institute of Virology", Dr. Ebright said "The documents make it clear that assertions by Dr. Collins and Dr. Fauci that the NIH did not support gain of function research are untruthful".

Almost no one else with that much to lose was willing to call out Drs. Fauci and Collins over the last two years. That's one of the reasons we're in the shape we're in now and we haven't seen the half of it yet.

Contrast Dr. Ebright's actions and comments regarding gain of function research with that of the of the authors of the "Proximal Origins" paper regarding the origin of the virus. All of them knew down deep that Fauci and Collins were lying when they claimed gain of function research was not being conducted in Wuhan and that the virus got into humans through natural zoonotic spillover. I don't work in this field and even I, was able to assess the likelihood that it arose from a bat or intermediate host. The likelihood was basically zero- I think it was 8 billion to one- and I said as much in my February 20, 2020 post, telling everyone I had proved the virus had human fingerprints all over it, i.e. that it came from a lab.

6. **Scott Jensen, M.D.**

Political enemies, far left Covidians, everyone went after Dr. Jensen but he hung tough in a state, Minnesota, that has veered strongly to the left in recent years.

7. **Simone Gold, M.D., J.D.**

She founded America's Front Line Doctors. Always willing to speak to a crowd and doesn't mince her words.

8. **Vladimir "Zev" Zelenko, M.D.**

We lost Dr. Zelenko earlier this year. He was a brave person in many ways and a pioneer in early treatment of SARS-2 infections.

9. **Peter Doshi, PhD**

Dr. Doshi would be sitting in the first seat on any committee I might chair regarding approval of treatments for public use. What a breath of fresh air! You must watch the following video. It shows this exceptional doctor giving testimony in a panel discussion sponsored by Senator Ron Johnson of Wisconsin. During his five minutes, Dr. Doshi put the relevant trial data on the screen behind him. Above the data was a quote by Drs. Walensky, Walke, and Fauci that read, "Clinical trials have shown that the vaccines authorized for use in the U.S. are highly effective against COVID-19 infection, severe illness and death." The date of that quote by Drs. Walensky et al was February 1, 2021. The vaccines had been going into arms for a month-and-a-half with the public under the impression that the vaccines were safe and effective in preventing infection, serious illness and death. Dr. Doshi then analyzed the data from the trials and said, "Those who claimed the trials showed the vaccines were effective in saving lives were wrong. The trials did not demonstrate this."

The point of this is not to show you yet another example of our government doctors lying to the public. The point is to show you a doctor who puts the data on the screen for all to see. We have had trouble getting those who supported the Narrative to show the data backing up their claims in an open debate. I challenged 16 medical doctors- most of them pediatricians in and around Jacksonville, Florida who had made their feelings clear and were in favor of childhood vaccine mandates, to a live debate as a public service. All declined. Steve Kirsch struck out, even when he offered anyone from the NIH, CDC or FDA $1 million for their time, to debate lockdowns, mask mandates, childhood vaccine mandates, etc. Please watch this video: https://www.youtube.com/watch?v=KL8SJRBNh_w

10. Peter Mc McCullough, M.D., MPH

Dr. McCullough was treating people very early and getting good results. His determination and commitment to proper treatment is admirable. He has paid a large price for his devotion to his patients and to the truth. He got released from his previous position at Baylor in Texas and now the Internal Medicine Board is threatening to pull his certification. It's ridiculous.

11. Pierre Kory, M.D.

Dr Kory is another person who has taken a lot of flak about the way he has (successfully) treated COVID-19 patients. He and Dr. Marek set up the FLCCC protocol that was used successfully by many doctors from all over the world. He has been perhaps the biggest proponent of the antiviral effects of IVM in COVID-19. Even the naysayers are starting to come around. The data are overwhelmingly in favor of its use in prophylaxis and treatment of COVID-19.

12. Ngozi Ezike, M.D.

This is a lady, a medical doctor, who thinks with her brain and feels with her heart.

Bravery? At the height of the early political tensions, the Democrats were trying to make Trump look as bad as possible. An easy way was to attribute as many deaths as possible to COVID-19 and accuse him of mismanagement.

In September of 2020, Dr Ezike stepped up to the microphone at a press conference as the Director of Public Health for the State of Illinois. Jay Pritzker, the liberal Governor of liberal Illinois, was standing behind her. She said, "Even if you died of a clear alternate cause of death but you had COVID at the same time, it's still listed as a COVID death. That means that everyone listed as a COVID death, it doesn't mean that was the *cause* of death but that they had COVID at the *time* of death. I hope that's helpful", and walked off the stage. Pritzker must have just about had a coronary.

13. Robert Malone, M.D., PhD

Dr. Malone was a pioneer in mRNA vaccine technology. He also knows a lot about how the three letter agencies and regulatory bodies operate.

14. Martin Kulldorff, PhD

Dr. Kulldorff is the only person who wrote the Stanford doctors that signed the letter denouncing Dr. Atlas. I'm sure he told them they were wrong and challenged all of them to debate the claims they made about Dr. Atlas. No one agreed. They were smart. They'd have no chance against Dr. Kulldorff. He has the facts on his side and he's brilliant. I requested an interview/discussion with him but I never heard back. There's still time. I want to run some of my ideas by him.

15. Jay Bhattacharya, M.D., PhD

Dr. Bhattacharya gave me 24 hours of long-form discussions over the spring months. We started out thinking we'd talk for an hour or so but there was so much to talk about, and we were enjoying it so much, we just kept going. We did a few sessions that went past the 8 hour mark. We started at 10 pm Phnom Penh time and didn't stop until after the sun came up the next morning. Dr. Bhattacharya and I had some disagreements. They made the videos very interesting and informative and I received lots of letters asking for more. The fact that I had never done any research and didn't know anything about epidemiology and public health actually helped the conversations go in directions you don't see very often.

One disagreement we had was whether asymptomatic transmission is possible. I insisted it was a first principles violation, meaning its existence would violate a fundamental principle having to do with the order in which a virus matures into its ability to go from human-to-human. A simple way to say it would be to ask the question: "How could you have asymptomatic transmission if it takes more viral load to enable human-to-human transmission than it does to create symptoms in the person spreading it?" What would be the implications if asymptomatic spread was possible?

To start with, we'd all be dead the first time we encountered a highly-contagious virus that also had a high mortality rate. It would also imply that people could die without ever having had symptoms. That would be a first principles violation too. Just imagine if small pox had the ability to spread without symptoms while carrying a 40% mortality rate. You wouldn't know who to avoid and half the people would be keeling over everywhere, without symptoms. It just doesn't make sense. Remember, someone who is PRE-symptomatic is not what we're talking about here. I don't have a first principles problem with that. So if your response is, "people could spread it around asymptomatically and to satisfy the 40% mortality requirement in your example, they would just get sick for a few days at some point and die. No. That would be a PRE symptomatic transmission which I have no problem with.

This was a real sticking point between Jay and me because Jay had data that showed asymptomatic transmission. I said, "Jay, there's got to be more to the story. Something is missing. This thing, as it stands is a first principles violation. It would violate everything we hold dear in logical thought." I thought and thought. How could both Jay and I be right? The answer is a little insertion into the SARS-2 genome called ORF-8. The ORF-8 gene produces a protein that blocks interferons from mediating symptoms. So these patients have the kinds of viral loads that allow transmission (which is more than enough to produce symptoms) but they experience no symptoms whatsoever.

This is the way the world could end and we as a society need to take every precaution to prevent it from happening. To start with, this type of gain of function should not just be discouraged, it should be BANNED.

There had to be something in the genome of the SARS-2 virus blocking symptoms in some patients with high viral loads. And I found that something in the knowledge databank of Dr. Stephen Quay during my discussions with him. This example shows one way in which previously unknown things are discovered. Something is wrong from a logical point of view. So you look for a previously-unknown entity that explains everything.

My first draft of this book contained a list that would have given readers a great example of how the practice of looking for an unknown helps one discover new things in science that just have to be there but I thought it superfluous since it was an example taken from physics.

I had made a list of physicians whom I considered "trial bound" to their detriment. I told the story of Albert Einstein- actually, any theoretical physicist would have worked- who used to sit in his chair and do thought experiments in his head, kind of like I just described in deriving fundamental contradictions if you assume asymptomatic transmission is possible. This is how Einstein came up with the general theory of relativity. He thought of experiments that would derive contradictions in the same way as I just described in showing you that asymptomatic spread cannot happen (without something like ORF-8) because if it could happen, something we know to be impossible could also happen. Therefore the original thing being considered, cannot happen. It's called "deriving a contradiction to prove your theory, false. We use this line of reasoning all the time in physics and mathematics and you should use it in your everyday life whenever you can.

The excellent Dr. Vinay Prasad was ranked #1 on this list. My ranking was based on a quote of Dr. Prasad's where he said something like, "right now, regarding lockdowns, there's no way to know if the benefits will outweigh the harms. Scientists will study this for the next ten years and the results of those studies will tell us." I wrote something cheeky like, "You don't have to go up on a roof with 100 bricks and drop them off to come to the conclusion that if you go up there next week and drop one off, it's going to go down, not up or sideways".

I was just trying to give some helpful advice to this very fine doctor. I want to see him think things through more, and not rely so much on trial results. It was just friendly advice. As Dr. Prasad's first instinct and Jay's too, in this case of asymptomatic transmission, was to look at the data to the detriment of reasoned thought. But this was a case where thinking it through was more beneficial; than even having rock-solid data "proving" its existence.

The point of bringing this up is that Einstein came up with a theory that was, in 1915, impossible to verify because we hadn't advanced technologically enough to check his theory by verifying, by measurement, its implications. We couldn't verify the gravitational red-shift of light, predicted by the General Theory for 40 years! When we finally measured it, it was the exact amount Einstein's theory predicted.

Another way to check the General Theory was by measuring Mercury's perihelion precession in its orbit about the sun; you know, the way a top precesses as it spins down. Well, this orbit had been measured and its precession was more than it should have been as predicted using Isaac Newton's Laws; roughly double what Newton predicted.

Not knowing anything about curved space-time (yet), the physicists of the day proposed a planet disturbing Mercury's orbit that was as yet undiscovered. They called it "Vulcan". It was never found, of course, Mercury's overly-precessing orbit was due to the curvature of space-time predicted by Einstein sitting in his rocking chair, thinking it through.

 Please appreciate how little the average star that is our sun perturbed the orbit by way of distorting space-time in the area of Mercury's orbit. The difference was only a few arc-seconds. An arc-second is 1/3600th of one degree, 360 of which make up a circle. The experimentalists measured that miniscule change in the orbit with telescopes from Earth's surface which itself, to me, anyway, is quite amazing. Here we are, eating macaroni and cheese and burning our feet on the asphalt parking lot at the beach because we forgot our shoes, yet we are able to measure a difference in the orbit of a little black dot moving across the surface of the sun compared to the last time it came around, to an accuracy of one part in 1,296,000 as we fly through the hollow of haze at 1.3 million miles an hour in our orbit around the sun which itself is orbiting around the center of mass of the Milky Way which, itself, is still exploding out from the Big Bang.

Just to tie a nice bow around this little tangent I took us on, the planet Neptune was discovered in the pitch darkness when the physicists at the time knew something had to be "out there" that was throwing Uranus's orbit off. They figured out where it should be, based on its affect on Uranus, and there it was.

Einstein's theory was complete, meaning, if any part of it could be proved wrong, all of it would have been wrong. Einstein was still living as experiment after experiment confirmed the General Theory of Relatively. When asked by a journalist how he might have felt if any of the experiments had not confirmed his theory, Einstein answered, "I would have felt bad for the Lord. The theory is correct."

The criminally destructive policies put in place for what, you will learn later, was close to a "nothing-burger", flies in the face of the beauty that is our universe and our place in it. We will recover from what was done to us. The human spirit will see to that.

After using a similar line of reasoning, I felt comfortable saying masks would not be able to block transmission of SARS-2 significantly, well before they were championed; just from reasoning from first principles. I describe my line of thought somewhere else in this book. I didn't need to see a single piece of data to figure that one out; lockdowns too. The point is, trials should be used to *confirm* theories we should be coming up with before a single trial participant signs up for the study. This is why I knew the Bangladesh trial had flaws when it "showed" some efficacy in wearing masks. When I finally looked at it, the flaw was glaringly obvious. There was bias in selecting people the villages being compared. Some people will sign up for a study just to get some freebies, in this case lots of colorful masks. If that's all they were looking for, they're going to be less likely to participate fully in the study. This makes it less likely they would, for example, report symptoms. Those pretty orange and pink masks are going to look a lot more effective than they really are if people don't return to report their symptoms

The world needs much more of the kind of dialogue I shared with Dr. Bhattacharya and requested once in a message to Dr. Prasad. Jay would certainly agree and that's probably one of the reasons he generously accepted without knowing me. I enjoyed watching him take a study apart when the authors went over the line in drawing conclusions. That's his forte.

16. Sunetra Gupta, PhD

When I presented a few of my ideas and proofs in graphic form to Dr. Bhattacharya during our 24 hours of videotaped discussions, and he said, "I think Sunetra Gupta would agree with you on this", he couldn't have paid me a higher compliment. She is commonly referred to as "the best epidemiologist in the world" by Drs. Kulldorff, Bhattacharya and many others. I wish she was more visible. She never fails to impress.

17. Steve Kirsch, MSEE

Let me first say that I've had problems getting through to Steve. He wrote me one time on Facebook messenger and asked me a question about immunology that I answered in great detail for him as I do for anyone. He never wrote me back after that, despite many attempts on my part. We were classmates at M.I.T. although we didn't know each other then. I don't understand why he has given me the cold shoulder. I must be missing something personal between Steve and me. But it doesn't matter. Steve belongs high on this very important list.

He's not a physician and it shows sometimes but he is a fine data analyst and he certainly would be considered a scientist by any fair-thinking person. He has an advanced degree in electrical engineering and computer science from M.I.T. which he tacked on to his undergraduate degree. He easily holds his own next to the others on this list but for slightly different reasons.

Steve is a spectacularly successful entrepreneur. He has built about 10 companies from the ground up. Remember when your computer mouse had a ball rolling around underneath it? It has a light now, doesn't it? Steve invented that, the optical mouse. Do you remember Infoseek, the early search engine? Steve started the company in 1993, just as things were getting started. It went public in 1996, the year it was the 5th most visited website on the net. Disney acquired it in 1999

Steve founded the COVID-19 Early Treatment Fund (CETF) at the beginning of the pandemic. He and CETF funded the research that showed promising results for fluvoxamine as an early treatment. Steve then founded the Vaccine Safety Research Foundation. It is a collaborative effort between Steve and a select group of scientists and doctors including Drs. Malone, McCullough, Bridle, Seneff, Rose and Bernstein. Their mission is to research the safety and efficacy of the vaccines and to keep the FDA as honest as they can.

Steve has also been generous with his money in offering $ 1 million to anyone from the CDC, NIH, or FDA if they would come and debate his group of experts on any of several topics where they differ. Steve will be happy for them to bring whomever they want to the debate. No one has taken him up as of September 12, 2022, which is shocking to me. I kind of (but not really) wish I was on the other side of the aisle from Steve on this one. My charity, Operation Kids, could use the million dollars.

I'm impressed but not the least bit surprised with what Steve has done in a field he wasn't familiar with at first. He has been a huge asset in exposing fraud in the vaccine trials and in real world data reporting by Big Pharma and their lackeys, the CDC, FDA, NIH, and mainstream Media.

18. John Lee, M.D.

Dr. Lee was very early and very correct.

19. Steven Quay, M.D., PhD

Dr. Quay knows as much about the molecular biology surrounding the origin of SARS-2 as anyone I can think of except, perhaps the people who put it together in the lab. He's working on a book about the origin. Look out for it.

Dr. Quay wears many hats. He is also conducting research on whether or not reducing the density of breast tissue will reduce the incidence of breast cancer. There is a strong correlation between tissue density as seen on mammogram and breast cancer risk.

20. Tess Lawrie, MBBCh, PhD

21. Andrew Bostom, M.D., M.S.

I saw testimony Dr. Bostom contributed to hearings in Rhode Island in which he explained how cases in the pediatric population were being exaggerated for nefarious purposes. He took a lot of flak from the ultra-woke Brown University where he worked and has been shunned by them. He was right, they were wrong. They should have championed him.

22. Ivor Cummins

Ivor was the first person to interview me. It was a case of "preaching to the choir" because we agreed on pretty much everything. Most of the presentation was me ripping through about 100 slides disproving what the experts were claiming. Our back and forth centered around the shock that no one else seemed to notice what we were seeing in the data, in particular, the experts. They were wrong about everything. There were others who understood things, of course, as I've come to learn; an amazing group from many walks of life who have mopped the floor with the so-called "experts". Ivor was front and center. He's a great data analyst and presents in a way that is understandable to the general public but not the slightest bit watered down. We talked for more than four hours over three days which I thought was a long time (until I hooked up with Bhattacharya).

Our video was wildly successful, garnering 65,000 views in a day-and-a-half. Then it was gone. YouTube pulled it.

23. Ryan Cole, M.D.

Pathologists know a lot of basic science as their job demands it; more, perhaps, than any other specialty. Dr. Cole is no exception. I try to tune in whenever I see he's being interviewed. He's another person with whom I wanted to do a long-form discussion. Without getting too technical, I wanted to run an idea I have by him about the spike protein's affect upon the regulation of ACE-2 receptors in light of ACE-2's antagonistic role toward angiotensin II in blood pressure control and inflammation. How does this compare quantitatively with the contribution of the spike protein's deleterious effects on vascular endothelium?

24. Mary Talley Bowden, M.D.

Dr. Bowden is suing Methodist Hospital of Houston, Texas for defamation, seeking $25 million. On November 12, 2021, Methodist made the mistake of posting claims about Dr. Bowden that were untrue, including that Dr. Bowden "is using her social media accounts to express her personal and political opinions about the COVID-19 vaccine and treatments." The statements from Houston Methodist continued, "These opinions, which are harmful to the community, do not reflect reliable medical evidence or the values of Houston Methodist, where we have treated more than 25,000 COVID-19 inpatients, and where all our employees and physicians are vaccinated to protect our patients," the hospital said. "Dr. Bowden, who has never admitted a patient at Houston Methodist Hospital, [and] is spreading dangerous misinformation which is not based in science."

Methodist was referring to statements made by Dr. Bowden that expressed her lack of support for vaccine mandates and eventually, for vaccines themselves because of the inability of the vaccines to block transmission, something that was well-known on November 12, 2021, when Methodist posted on social media.

I know a lot about this issue because I was the first to prove the vaccines weren't blocking transmission. I had suspected they wouldn't block transmission before they were released on December 14, 2020. Then, in mid-January, I had enough case data (out of Israel) to feel certain I was right.

I referred to my findings in a video explaining this on January 24, 2021. It took the general medical community at least until April to acknowledge this because my videos were getting only about 1000 views each, possibly due to shadow banning by YouTube. Drs. Fauci and Walensky did not realize it until at least June and President Biden until at least August of 2021. It's not clear whether or not he knows this even today, although he recently contracted COVID-19 after two doses and two boosters.

It's surprising that Houston Methodist's CEO, Dr. Marc Boom would OK a statement like, "all our employees and physicians are vaccinated to protect our patients." It appears Houston Methodist is the one "spreading dangerous misinformation which is not based in science." At the time this statement was posted, it was admitted, even by Drs. Fauci and Walensky, that the vaccines were not capable of blocking transmission. Implying that they *were*, gave people a false sense of security and thus, this misinformation was and is dangerous.

25. Paul Marik, M.D.

26. Byram Bridle, PhD

Canada's hero. I have one bone to pick with him. It was I who was the first to raise concerns that the vaccine would most likely travel to distant sites in the body after being injected into the recipient's deltoid muscle. I did so before the vaccines came out. The Japanese study Dr. Bridle so alertly brought to the attention of the world, appeared after the vaccine campaign was well underway. YouTube may have shadow-banned me down to 500 views, but I had learned by then to take screenshots! Just kidding. Nobody cares who was first, except, of course, the person who was first. It was yet another Kafka-esque, "Old Man and the Sea" experience for me; a nightmare I still haven't woken up from. We'll see how well this book sells.

27. Aaron Kheriaty, M.D.

28. Dr. Clare Craig

29. Dr. Wolfgang Wodarg

30. Richard Urso, M.D.

31. Ron Paul, M.D., R-TX

Dr. Paul has an internet show called "The Liberty Report". Without making a big show of it, he's been right about everything, at least as far as I can tell from the many installments I've seen. I can't believe we never elected him President. Imagine if we'd had a medical doctor with Dr. Paul's smarts at the helm during COVID-19, instead of, for example, Joe Biden, who said, ten months after we knew otherwise, "If you get vaccinated, you won't get sick". Dr. Paul would have gotten a lot of things right for us; not just COVID-19.

10 *M.D. Bureaucrats Who Continue to Get It Terribly Wrong*

1. Anthony Fauci, M.D.
2. Deborah Birx, M.D.
3. Rochelle Wallensky, M.D.
4. Ashish Jha, M.D., MPH

Dr. Jha was picked by President Biden on March 17, 2022 to takeover as COVID-19 Response Coordinator . On June 20, 2022, he said the vaccines were safe and effective and urged parents to vaccinate their six-month to 5-year-olds. How could someone say this after all we know about myocarditis and other significant and dangerous side effects such as anaphylaxis and Guillian-Barre syndrome? This doctor has been off the mark on just about everything since the beginning of this but keeps getting invited on Good Morning America, CNN, MSNBC, The NBC Evening News, etc. This is because he tows the political/Big Pharma narrative. He just skims the surface on everything. He has no depth of understanding. When he does venture into explaining something, he gets it completely wrong. Here is the way he justifies this nonsense. "My take is people are not looking for certainty. People are looking for judgment", said Dr. Jha. "And it's fine to give judgment as long as you're not overstating the data." But, Dr. Jha, it's not fine to give judgment when that judgment does not correspond to the data in any way.

5. Peter Marks, M.D. PhD

Director of the Center for Biologics Evaluation and Research at the FDA. He is concerned about vaccine hesitancy by parents for their 6 months to 11-year-old children. He recommends that they be vaccinated with an experimental treatment that does not protect them from getting or transmitting the virus and about which we do not know the long term side effects. The trials used too few people. Neither the vaccinated group nor the control group showed any serious disease or side effects in the few months they followed them. Not at all surprising for a disease where around a million children this age would have had to get infected before one died. They only used a few thousand in the trials. To determine the efficacy of the vaccine, antibody levels were checked and compared to older age groups, even adults, from previous trials. Comparisons are made and a level is chosen above which the child is considered protected. This is followed by vaccinating all of the controls so there is no matched group to which they can be compared in the future. The trial designers will say that they vaccinate the controls to protect the participants but they're really doing it to protect the vaccine makers.

6. Francis Collins, M.D., PhD
7. Leanna Wen, M.D.
8. Tom Frieden, M.D., MPH
9. Robert Redfield, M.D.
10. Scott Gotlieb, M.D.

15 *Women Responsible for the Most Death and Destruction*

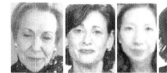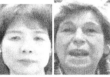

1. Deborah Birx, M.D.

One of the most vocal and, as White House Advisor, powerful proponents of lockdowns, the most egregious public health policy in history, was Dr. Birx. She will be remembered for her refusal to listen to the other side of the argument.

On top of what all that means in terms of the death and destruction of innocent people, she managed to mislead the people about the vaccines as well. She offered this comment recently: "I knew these vaccines were not going to protect against infection. And I think we overplayed the vaccines." You KNEW the vaccines weren't going to block transmission and you didn't speak up? Do you think, maybe, some people's risk/benefit analysis would change, knowing the vaccines didn't protect them from getting infected? This is worse than her pushing lockdowns that will, according to the WHO, result in 140 million deaths from starvation.

She could plead stupidity for not knowing lockdowns were a horrible idea. But knowing before they were released (according to her), the vaccines weren't going to block transmission, while Drs. Fauci and Walensky were on TV for 7+ months saying if you've had the vaccine, you can't get infected, putting innocent people at increased risk of infection because of false security, she definitely contributed to the deaths of innocent people in this way too; that is, if she's telling the truth.

It turns out, Dr. Birx claiming she knew the vaccines were not going to block transmission is just revisionist history. I found a quote from December of 2020 that contradicts what she's claiming now She is on record as saying, "This is one of the most highly-effective vaccines we have in our infectious disease arsenal. And so that's why I'm very enthusiastic about the vaccine".

She was also completely fooled by the fake propaganda videos released to the world by China in January of 2020 (Please see **3 Reasons Why We Can Be Sure There Was Planning Beforehand**"). She still goes all gushy praising the "courageous" Chinese doctor who notified the world of this "horrific" new disease. In her book, released in April, 2022, she writes, "The video showed a hallway crowded with patients slumped in chairs. Some of the masked people leaned against the wall for support. The camera didn't pan so much as zigzag while the Chinese doctor maneuvered her smart phone up the narrow corridor. My eye was drawn to two bodies wrapped in sheets lying on the floor amid the cluster of patients and staff. The doctor's colleagues, their face shields and other personal protective equipment in place, barely glanced at the lens as she captured the scene. They looked past her, as if at a harrowing future they could all see and hoped to survive. I tried to increase the volume, but there was no sound. My mind seamlessly filled that void, inserting the sounds from my past, sounds from other wards, other places of great sorrow." Sure, there's enough melodrama there to put "As the World Turns" to shame but she believes it.

The stupidity associated with this thing is mind boggling.

Or maybe not...

Mind Boggling... I've said that many times but, now, I'm beginning to think all of this – ALL OF THIS FROM THE VERY BEGINNING-might have been years in the making. I'm talking everything. What if everything you've seen or read, down to the tiniest detail was part of a grand plan to rob the middle classes of their money and power to rearrange the way civilization is organized. The amount of money stolen to date has already been calculated to be $3.8 trillion in the U.S. alone.

Consider this line of speculation: They got the idea from the SARS-1 outbreak. They would have to wait until the technology caught up with their plans. Suddenly all systems were go. They could create any virus they wanted in a lab. We've been able to order whatever genome segments we want from a commercial catalog for years and they're cheap. All they had to do was stick them together on a coronavirus backbone. Science fiction had become reality.

Every detail... From the miners who died in 2012 cleaning guano (that they could never find the causative organism for. Hell. I could have isolated the causative organism and I've never stepped foot in a lab), to the fake videos of people collapsing in the streets of Wuhan (to show you how horrible the disease is, the disease that is coming for YOU (so you better do what we say), to the city-wide fountain parties in Wuhan, shortly after the lockdowns finished, the pictures of which conveniently appeared on the internet to show everyone in the world how well the lockdowns worked, convincing enough to fool a world of terrified people into giving up their livelihoods, health insurance and life savings and agree to the most idiotic public health policy in history, turning negative, every GDP in the world, except for China's, of course, which actually ended the year up 3.5% while rerouting all of the shipping lanes in the world to their benefit.

Sure, it's speculation- even wild speculation, but I can't get around the fact that explains *everything*.

I sometimes imagine a scene in the Women's Room at an undisclosed location between Deborah Birx and Susan Wojcicki.

EXTERIOR-DAY
Stationary drone shot from above. A rectangular, concrete block BUILDING, surrounded by thick pine forest. The words "Somewhere in Northern China" appear on the screen and fade out.

An industrial, dated, circa 1950s women's BATHROOM- INTERIOR-DAY

A close up of a lady's hand removing a brown paper towel from a dispenser. She has an expensive bracelet on and finely polished nails. Her hand appears middle-aged. She brings the paper towel down and places it between her finger and the soap dispenser button (to keep from touching it) and squirts soap into her other hand. She throws the paper towel into a tall, gray, opaque waste paper receptacle nearby.

DEBORAH Birx is washing her hands at the sink, lingering. SUSAN Wojcicki comes out of a stall and goes to the adjacent sink to wash her hands. Deborah nods. Susan nods back.

> DEBORAH
> What's your name?
> SUSAN
> S.M.W.N. ...
> DEBORAH (interjects)
> Cut the crap. What's your real name?
> I've been sitting next to you for three
> days in there. I can't take this anymore.

Deborah smiles at Susan. Susan cups her ear and sweeps her hand around the room, then shrugs her shoulders as if to ask, "What about bugs?"

> DEBORAH
> Forget it. These people are
> CINOs, Communists In Name Only. In
> actuality, they're PWSOWSCs. Sorry,
> Progressive Wokester Straight Outta

Wall Street Capitalists. What would it
look like if they got caught bugging the
ladies room? Sorry about the initialisms,
old medical school habit. What's your
name?

                    SUSAN (nods)
            Susan.

They start to shake and abort because their hands are soapy. They touch elbows awkwardly with a
giggle, as if they just learned how.

                    SUSAN
        You?
                    DEBORAH
        Deborah. Deb.
                    SUSAN
         You're in...?
                    DEBORAH
        White House medical..." (Susan
        nods in approval) Trump manipulation.
                    SUSAN
        You, not TNTIDD81?
                    DEBORAH
        No way. Trump's an old horn-dog.
        They needed a woman. (Susan nods) What
        about you? (Susan looks confused) Why...
        are... you... here?

                    SUSAN (chuckles while looking at Deborah):
            Oh...Censorship. (reaches for a paper towel to dry her hands)
            I run YouTube.
 Deborah is reaching for a paper towel while nodding with surprised approval, pausing, as Susan
removes hers)
                    DEBORAH
        Not bad.
    -Cut to-
The ladies are facing each other drying their hands.

                    DEBORAH
        You know the guy who spoke after... what's his
        name... 'Big Creepy' this morning?
                    SUSAN
        Yeah, that's a good name for him.
        I couldn't understand a word he said.

(imitates Klaus Schwab in English with
a thick German accent to chuckles from
both women). You mean that
smokestack who was a (shows fingers
making inverted commas) journalist over
here (adding, with an incredulous look
on her face) before being granted an age
waiver and enlisting in the Marines?
                    DEBORAH
Yeah, that's him.
(whispers to Susan) He recruited me.
                    SUSAN (excited)
Wow, you know that guy?
                    DEBORAH
Not before all this. He's the Head of the White
House Group. I knew his wife. We worked together
at the CDC... Yeah, he's a 'Raftie' alright.
                    SUSAN (looking confused at first)
Oh, I get it; another acronym. What does it mean?
                    DEBORAH
First of all, it's an initialism, not an acronym. The
letters don't spell a word. Second, It doesn't
mean anything. Initialisms and acronyms *stand*
for something. Anyway, in this case, 'Raftie' is
neither. It's a *descriptive* term, for a... a hunk with
a brain. You know... if your plane goes down? You
want to share a raft with *him*... in case you end up
on a desert island for the rest of your lives
and have to repopulate the world... (winks at
Susan)
                    SUSAN (glassy-eyed, nods, as she says):
Yeah.(detached, as if imagining it.)

The two ladies toss their paper towels into the trash can and walk toward the door.

                    DEBORAH
Hey, him recruiting me and all, his wife.... That's on the
Q.T. (Susan looks confused.) It's an old Latin
Term, 'quietus-something' another tip for ya, if you ever want to
go to medical school, learn some Latin. It means
'For your ears only', capiche?
                    SUSAN
Wouldn't that be a *phrase,* instead of a *term*?
It's two words. (looks at Deborah for approval)

DEBORAH (rolling her eyes upward):
Whatever.
Deborah is looking straight ahead as she gets a cigarette out, lights it and takes a puff)
DEBORAH
You know, in this business, you gotta learn to keep your
mouth, shut. Capiche?
SUSAN (head down, appearing dejected at not
impressing Deborah with the 'phrase' vs.
'term' distinction, answers softly with her head
down):
Sure. (corrects herself immediately) Capiche.
(looks up at Deborah with a 'don't hit me' expression)
DEBORAH (looking disapprovingly down at Susan):
Greenhorns.

Deborah points at the door with an open hand.

DEBORAH
Well?

Susan nods and starts for the door. Deborah stops her.

DEBORAH
You use 'em too, you know; initialisms.
SUSAN
What do you mean?
DEBORAH
You just called him TNTIDD.
SUSAN
Yeah, I know. That's Dr. Fauci's code name, right?
DEBORAH (looking very frustrated with
Susan now):
Didn't I just tell you, you gotta learn to keep your
mouth shut? Never mention someone's real name,
especially in the same sentence, with their code name.
Got it?
SUSAN (apologetic)
Oh gosh. Sorry.

Susan turns and heads toward the door to go out. Deborah stops her again.

DEBORAH
The initialism. You know what it means?
SUSAN
You mean Fauci's

32

code name? It *means* something?

DEBORAH (looking very frustrated at Susan's use of Fauci's real name again)
For the last time, it doesn't *mean* anything. It *stands* for something. Ok?

SUSAN
Oh yeah. What does it stand for?

DEBORAH
The Nation's Top Infectious Disease Doctor'. He came up with it... "

SUSAN
Really?

DEBORAH (sarcastically)
All by himself.

SUSAN
Wow, that's cool. (cut to Deborah's face, looking incredulously at Susan) I always wondered what it would feel like to be the best at something. You know, the top person, like Tiger Woods in golf or Anthony Fau I mean TNTIDD81 in infectious disease doctoring. Do you think they would let me make up my own code name?

DEBORAH:
That would be a big fat 'No'. Tell me something, Susan. How do you run a multi-billion dollar company?" (Susan takes in a big breath like she's going to answer the question but Deborah interrupts), "Never mind." (points at door)

Susan turns and goes out the door. Deborah stands alone, looking off into the distance, nodding. After a few more puffs of her cigarette, she drops it on the floor and stamps it out with the sole of her shoe, looks in the full-length mirror by the door, adjusts her bra and then her scarf, waits a few counts with her hand on the door handle opening it and going out.
-CUT TO-
HALLWAY of the non-descript building- INTERIOR-DAY
Deborah walks 30 feet behind Susan as several people pass them, glancing at the two ladies without moving their heads and without nodding in recognition.

-FADE OUT-
Large OFFICE-INTERIOR-NIGHT

Xi JINPING, KLAUS Schwab, BILL Gates, FRANCES Collins, ANTHONY Fauci, SECRETARY, TRANSLATOR 1, TRANSLATOR 2 and four MILITARY GUARDS are standing in a very large office, exquisitely decorated and furnished. Two Guards each stand aside the two entrances to the room. The two translators are standing to the side in view of Xi Jinping, together, away from the central focus of Xi, Schwab, and Gates. Collins and Fauci are standing outside the circle but close enough to be involved in the conversation.
-CUT TO-
METAL DETECTOR-INTERIOR-NIGHT
Susan is going through a metal detector located in the lobby of the same building, staffed by six Chinese military guards and four technicians. She picks up a briefcase as it comes through the scanner and hurries down the hallway toward the interior of the building.
-CUT TO-
HALLWAY-INTERIOR-NIGHT
Susan hurries up to a non-descript door and enters some numbers into her phone. She touches a fingerprint scanner on her phone's screen
-CUT TO-
Large OFFICE-INTERIOR-NIGHT
A red light illuminates over a door as a pleasant tone sounds. The door opens and Susan enters. Jinping looks at her without changing expression. Everyone stops talking. No one greets her, nor her, them. She walks over to a table as if she is familiar with the surroundings. Everyone is crowded around her as she enters the code and releases the latches on the briefcase.

-CUT TO-
CONTROL ROOM INT/NIGHT
MATTHEW Pottinger is sitting in a small CONTROL ROOM looking intently at a monitor. The screen glow reflects on his face.

-CUT TO monitor feed-
The resolution is poor. Susan takes what appears to be recording equipment from the briefcase and turns it on. It is clear from Susan's movements that a recording is being played but there is no sound coming through the monitor.

-CUT TO-
MATTHEW's face in the monitor glow

.

■ To be continued…

2. Rochelle Walensky, M.D.
Her very poor advice to vaccinate small children when trial data provided absolutely no justification for it was far outside the bounds of ethical behavior by a medical doctor. Amoral or immoral; take your pick. We'll probably never know whether or not she knew what she was doing was wrong but

that's no excuse. Along with Dr. Birx, another person who had trouble understanding the science, she misled the public over and over again on issues as important as knowing whether or not the vaccines blocked transmission. At least five months after it was known that they did not, she was saying publicly that vaccinated persons constituted "dead ends" for the virus. This was done out of ignorance or in an attempt to sell more vaccines to an unwary public; the former landing her in the unemployment line, the latter in prison. She also withheld data from the public that could have helped them decide whether or not to get these horrible injections.

When Robert Redfield was replaced by Rochelle Walensky, I and many others were hoping for an improvement over Redfield who was so clueless, he once held up a surgical mask in Senate testimony and said, "Face coverings are the most powerful public health tool the nation has against the coronavirus and might even provide better protection against it than a vaccine."

"We have clear scientific evidence they work, and they are our best defense," Dr. Redfield added. "I might even go so far as to say that this face mask is more guaranteed to protect me against Covid than when I take a Covid vaccine that is 70% effective."

This bizarre claim was made by Dr Redfield on September 28, 2020 when he and everyone else assumed the vaccine would function like we have come to expect vaccines to function; blocking transmission in particular, so recipients could have some degree of confidence that after they got the injections, they would be protected from getting the disease. No one knew at that time- before the vaccine rollout- that the mRNA "vaccines" would not work like vaccines at all; failing to block transmission, etc. I did make a post on December 4, 2020, before the vaccine administration had begun, where I speculated that the vaccines were not going to block transmission. As I have said already, I proved this on January 15, 2021, about a month after the December 14 rollout. Nevertheless Drs. Fauci and Walensky continued telling the public that the vaccines *did* block infection, well into July of 2021. The M.D.T.V. Mafia chimed in as did show hosts on Leftist Media outlets such as CNN and MSNBC, Rachel Maddow being the most visible because of her superior communications skills, a close-to-ideal propaganda kill machine.

Dr. Walensky strongly supported masks, lockdowns, and vaccines and was very late in getting schools reopened, causing profound, lifelong harm to affected children. After knowing the risks of death in small children, she actively promoted the vaccination of toddlers and babies down to six months of age without adequate safety and efficacy data even though it was well-known that the chance of a healthy child in this age group dying from COVID-19 was on the order of one person in a million. Note that a six month old child cannot walk or talk and Dr. Walensky promoted vaccines to their new parents with absolutely no justification.

3. Leana Wen, M.D.

Dr. Wen is the former President of Planned Parenthood. Aside from Deborah Birx, she was the strongest proponent of lockdowns. From her enormous platform on CNN, she appeared almost daily, pushing deadly policies like lockdowns, mask use by the general public and vaccines. Even after omicron hit, she continued to push for mandates of a vaccine and boosters made for the original strain when the data was clear. The vaccines increased overall mortality in recipients. Dr. Wen (after Omicron was circulating): "We should mandate proof of vaccination — and boosters — for all indoor dining, gyms, movie theaters, and sporting events." In this quote she is pushing for vaccine mandates.

Could she be so stupid as to not realize some people have gotten the disease and recovered from it? They don't need a vaccine, especially one that doesn't work and increases your chance of dying.

Also, she's ignoring people with immunity-in-place. That's about 40% of the population and they shouldn't get a vaccine either; even one that worked! She probably knows this, so she's pushing for vaccine mandates for another reason. It certainly has nothing to do with helping or protecting people. When she wrote out this opinion on Linkedin, it had been more than a year since we knew the vaccines did not prevent a recipient from getting or spreading the disease. So why vaccinate? It doesn't stop the spread and increases your chance of dying from all causes. On top of all this, she doesn't understand why giving vaccines that don't prevent spread, while an active pandemic is occurring, puts selective pressure on emerging variants.

She also pushed masks after 74 years of meta-analyses of randomized, controlled trials showed they didn't reduce transmission significantly. If she couldn't understand why masks didn't work, she should have looked at the literature. A leading member of the M.D.T.V. Mafia, she was wrong and continues to be wrong on virtually every call.

Recently, as political winds have shifted, Dr. Wen has changed her tune on lockdowns. This has put her out of favor with the far-Left "Covidians". They removed her from some committees and cancelled a few of her speaking engagements. Dr. Wen has received some favorable press and sympathy for changing her stance on lockdowns and for the mistreatment she has suffered at the hands of those far Leftists in control of her appearances and committees.

Journalist Jeffrey Tucker was very easy on Dr. Wen in a recent piece about her softening on the lockdowns she pushed so vigorously; apparently overlooking the fact that those lockdowns have sent and will send many millions of innocent people, including children, to their deaths. I agree with Jeffrey on most of the things he writes- almost all, actually- but I disagree on this one. Should we let the perpetrators go free or even be praised for "coming around" as if nothing happened when the truth is that at least 150 million innocent people will die because of the policies those perpetrators pushed? When someone in prison "comes around" to being against murder, does he get released or does his punishment continue? To put it in perspective, consider that the number of deaths we're talking about here amount to more than two times the number caused by Hitler, Stalin, and Mao, *combined*.

4. Susan Wojcicki

The YouTube CEO's censoring activities prevented millions of people from accessing information that could have saved their lives and those of their family members. The meta-analyses showing the efficacy of ivermectin and hydroxychloroquine showed that their use could have prevented millions of deaths had YouTube not blocked this knowledge from the general public. See "13 Most Prolific Censors".

5. Shi Zheng Li

She has slipped by so far, for the most part, but when the truth is finally revealed in full, she, along with Ralph Baric and Peter Daszak are going to be found to have been the actual creators of the SARS-2 virus. I'm speculating a little here. I don't like to say things I can't prove and this has held me in good stead so far, so I do have to qualify this somewhat. I haven't worked out all of the details yet, but I have plenty of reasons to think I'm right.

Daszak did the field work with bats in the Yunnan caves (see Appendix II). Baric was the technical virtuoso who shared critical technology such as the method for reverse-engineering spike proteins, producing the model upon which various prototypes were tested to see if the spike proteins so-created could get into human pneumocytes (and actually sent humanized mice to Dr Shi to use when her lab at the Wuhan Institute of Virology couldn't quite work out the details to make it happen). At the Wuhan Institute of Virology, Dr Shi was able to freely conduct the unacceptable gain of function research enabling asymptomatic transmission and inhibition of the human immunological response , at that time under moratoria in the U.S. and strongly frowned upon internationally.

Dr. Si in particular, has done some very suspicious things so far. In a Scientific American interview, she lied about the causative organism in the death of miners in Mojiang, Yunnan in 2012. She said the pneumonia the miners suffered from with three of the six eventually dying, after cleaning bat guano from a copper mine, was of *fungal* origin. This does happen sometimes, but in this case, a PhD graduate student had already published his thesis about the case, in which he demonstrates clearly using radiological evidence that the pneumonia was caused by the virus. How could Dr. Shi not knowing something that important having poured over the victims' charts and discussing this in detail with every expert she could find? The answer is, Dr. Shi could not have known that the pneumonia that killed those miners was of viral origin. There's no way she didn't know this. She and her team visited the caves located 1100 miles away, where the miners were working, no less than 13 times to collecting 1322 samples to take back to the lab in Wuhan for sequencing and analysis. Almost 300 corona viruses were found in those samples; nine beta corona viruses, the same subgroup from which SARS-1 and SARS-2 come. Why would she do all that work to find viruses if she thought the pneumonia was caused by a fungus? It seems the more important question is, "Why did she lie about the causative agent to Scientific American?

That PhD thesis, by the way, was found by searching the Chinese internet by someone in India. A detailed study about a mystery virus that killed half of the people infected with it- something this incredibly important- had never been translated into English; a *2016* PhD thesis, in this day and age after SARS-1 in 2003 and Swine flu in 2009 and 2010??

The other thing that struck me as unusual, was that the causative organism was never disclosed; that I could find.

That PhD graduate student, Huang Canping worked under George Gao, the Director of the Chinese CDC who is quoted as saying at the Gates Foundation/Johns Hopkins U./World Economic Forum-sponsored in October of 2019, "

Combine all of this with a completely off the wall quote she delivered when interviewers asked a few too many questions, "

She changed the name of the virus that killed the miners cleaning the bat caves in Mojiang province in 2013 RaTG13) and lied in a Scientific American interview, claiming the pneumonia those miners got was a fungal pneumonia. All of the medical records and x-rays showed it was a viral pneumonia and she was aware of that. Also, she authored one of the 14 papers dealing with the insertion of a Furin cleavage site genome into a viral RNA backbone after years of collaborating with Ralph Baric of UNC who did much of the original work and who sent humanized mice to Wuhan for use by Dr Shi at the Wuhan Institute of Virology.

6. Randi Weingarten

Ms. Weingarten is the President of the National Federation of Teachers, the second largest teacher union in the U.S. It's a real eye-opener to read the emails she sent to the CDC. When you add up the life-years lost in children who had their education disrupted, in light of Ms. Weingarten's push to keep schools closed (providing her union members their full salary while not working), she pops up to #6 on this list. The Democratic Party, the teachers Unions, one of which is presided over by Ms Weingarten, and the leftist media weren't going to let the well-being of children get in the way of making Trump look bad. The school shutdowns will result in this group of students dropping out more often, earning less and dying earlier than if school closures had not stayed in place so long, compliments of Ms. Weingarten. Ordinary teachers for the most part, didn't speak out when they learned about the damage being done to children by Ms. Weingarten. Disgraceful.

7. Theresa Tam

Dr. Tam is the Chief Public Health Officer of Canada. She claims Canada would have had 800,000 deaths if lockdowns hadn't been put in place. Canada has had 43,158 deaths "because of" and "with" COVID. There is no evidence anywhere that lockdowns prevented deaths and tons of evidence that they did nothing significant.

8. Rachel Maddow

I don't get MSNBC overseas where I am but I've seen enough clips on YouTube of Ms. Maddow proclaiming, (paraphrasing) if you get the vaccine, you can't get the virus and you can't send it on to someone else. She made dozens of statements like this during the initial vaccine rollout in 2021. If believed and acted upon- and there's no reason to think they wouldn't be-these statements were enough to kill hordes and hordes of people.

Here's an exact quote; this one from March 21, 2021: "The virus stops with every vaccinated person. A vaccinated person gets exposed to the virus, the virus does not infect them. The virus cannot then use that person to go anywhere else. It cannot use a vaccinated person as a host to get other people." Rachel was making false statements about the transmission of the SARS-2 virus; statements that, if believed, and acted upon, most certainly resulted in the deaths of innocent people; lots and lots of them. This particular statement was aired months after I proved the vaccines in fact, did NOT block transmission. Rachel may not have known the truth. In March, people educated in this field- epidemiologists, medical doctors, data analysts- were still telling me I couldn't possibly have figured it out that fast, that there hadn't been enough data released by then. But there had been, if you understood the implications of immunity-in-place.

Could Rachel Maddow have figured it out? No. Could she have understood it if I had explained it to her? I don't know. But that's no excuse. If Rachel didn't know anything about this subject, she should not have commented on it; not when people's lives were and are at stake. Do you think any children have died because their parents got them vaccinated after seeing this?

To further elucidate Rachel Maddow's lack of understanding of this virus and disease, consider the following statement made by her, also in March of 2021, when the vaccine rollout was just beginning to find its legs: "We need to vaccinate as many people as possible as fast as possible, really, as suddenly as possible, to prevent the emergence and circulation of the variants. Is that fair?" to which Rochelle Walensky, the CDC Director and ranked #2 on this list, replied, "You are exactly right", which in itself is shocking in its display of ignorance of the risks involved in vaccinating a population during an ongoing pandemic with a vaccine that does not block transmission.

Maddow's statement, of course, is the exact opposite of reality. IT IS EXACTLY THE OPPOSITE. Giving vaccines that do not block transmission during an active pandemic is the very reason why strong variants emerge. The so-called "leaky" vaccines exert selective pressure on the process of variant emergence. The knowledge that the vaccines don't block transmission coupled with the knowledge that we reached herd immunity to the Wuhan strain both demonstrated by me before January 15, 2021, should make you understand the destructive and deadly impact of censorship by YouTube in particular but social media companies in general. The truth about the virus and vaccines was kept from the public. Meanwhile, people like Rachel Maddow were recklessly spewing false and dangerous nonsense about the vaccines with wonton disregard for the lives of millions of innocent people.

It makes you wonder if there was ever any reason to get vaccinated. The vaccines didn't protect the recipient from getting infected. They didn't help us reach herd immunity. They increased our risk of dying from a myriad of other diseases. OK, but the trials showed they helped prevent serious illness and death from COVID-19, right? Not according to Peter Doshi. (please see *"Physicians/Scientists Most Brave in Fighting the Narrative"*)

9. Brianna Keilar

The CNN host is one of the worst offenders at CNN. I'll just give you one example. In January of 2022, Joe Rogan had an Australian TV and radio broadcaster on his show named Josh Szeps. Szeps claimed that a person is about eight times more likely to get myocarditis from COVID-19 than from the vaccines in young people. This surprised Rogan who remembered differently, thinking the vaccines caused more myocarditis so he asked his assistant to look it up. The assistant looked it up and found evidence that Szeps was correct. But the assistant made a serious error when he looked it up. He didn't limit the search to young people as Rogan specified and he limited his answer to the Pfizer vaccine only. Pfizer's vaccine is not anywhere near as bad when it comes to causing myocarditis as Moderna's. More on the actual facts below.

Brianna Keilar did a show about how Rogan was spreading false information, based on this interview disagreement with Szeps. She had a guest on, a lady epidemiologist named Katrine Wallace who had signed a letter with 250 other people that read, "By allowing the propagation of false and societally harmful assertions, Spotify [Spotify bought Rogan's catalog of past podcasts and he posts new ones there (all for $100 million)] is enabling its hosted media to damage public trust in scientific research and sow doubt in the credibility of data-driven guidance offered by medical professionals." Those people were lobbying to have Rogan removed from Spotify for supposedly remembering something wrong and looking it up on the air! Keilar used the interview with Szeps to claim Rogan was spreading false information because he first thought the opposite of what the guest claimed. So Rogan had his assistant look it up. Is there anyone reading this who is not mentally ill who considers that spreading false information? Of course not. It's exactly what a person with journalistic integrity should do. CNN should take a lesson from it.

Kevlar's guest said, "a podcast of the size that Joe Rogan has and the effect of misinformation spreading to such a large audience, they have sort of a responsibility to the public during a public health emergency to protect the public from this kind of misinformation and harmful information going to the public and right now we have 26% of our population that is still unvaccinated and misinformation like this directly contributes to that." The epidemiologist too, thinks that not remembering something and looking it up constitutes spreading misinformation!

I've got some news for Brianna Keilar, the epidemiologist Katrine Wallace, the Australian broadcaster Josh Szeps and Rogan's assistant. Rogan was right in the cohort he clearly specified, "young people". Here's the data to prove it:

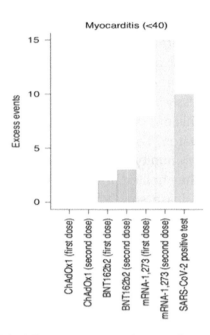

Myocarditis (<40)

BNT is Pfizer. mRNA is the Moderna vaccine. The positive SARS-2 group ("getting it from the disease") is on the right in pink. Moderna's bar is 50% higher after the second dose, the definition of being vaccinated at that time. I'm being conservative by letting "young people" go up to 40 years of age. 40 is considered middle aged, not young. What if we defined young people as being, say, below 25? The Moderna bars would be much, much higher, relative to the SARS-2 positive bar.

Expected vs. Observed reports after Pfizer-BioNTech dose 2, 7-day risk period (N=549)*

Age group, years	Females		Males	
	Cases of myopericarditis, expected	Cases of myopericarditis, observed	Cases of myopericarditis, expected	Cases of myopericarditis, observed
12–15*	0–3	12	1–5	116
16–17*	0–2	15	0–3	120
18–24*	0–5	11	1–7	134
25–29*	0–4	4	1–5	30
30–39	1–13	7	1–11	40
40–49	1–13	12	1–11	26
50–64	2–22	9	2–19	5
65+	2–22	4	2–18	4

* As of Aug 18, 2021; assumes a 7-day observation window; with 549 of 765 reports after mRNA vaccines occurring during Days 0–6 after vaccination; counts among 12–29 years from reports meeting case definition for myopericarditis; expected estimates for females 12–29 years adjusted to reflect reduced incidence in this age group   8

Look at the last table. It was supplied by the CDC. In both females and males- especially males- below the age of 25, after dose 2, the numbers of myocarditis are astronomical compared to what is expected in non-vaccinated for each age group. And this is for the Pfizer vaccine. The Moderna numbers are about five times higher!

Now you can see what being young really means as far as risk of getting myocarditis after these vaccines is concerned. For late teens up to age 25, the risk is much, much higher from the vaccines than from the disease. Many countries have banned Moderna vaccines from being used in young men because the risk of myocarditis is so high. It's not a benign disease. Almost half of the heart transplants done in the U.S. are because of myocarditis.

Who was wrong here? Brianna Keilar was wrong. Rogan's assistant was wrong and screwed up massively. Josh Szeps (who I heard called Rogan to apologize for correcting him when he (Rogan) was right). The 250 who signed the letter if this was part of the reason for writing it were wrong. Finally, the epidemiologist, Katrine Wallace was wrong by signing the letter and she was wrong based on what she said on Keilar's show. Talk about spreading misinformation! How could she not know something this important in her own field? And then to go on national TV and not even look it up beforehand? On top of that, she was pushing those horrible vaccines. This was in January of 2022! That is a year after we knew they didn't block transmission and there were all kinds of data available that showed they damage your immune system and cause far more deaths from other causes than they might save from COVID-19! Please watch the video knowing what you now know about myocarditis. https://www.youtube.com/watch?v=X4oRlqPntY8&t=26s

10. Gretchen Whitmer

Required that nursing homes accept patients infected with the SARS-2 virus, resulting in the deaths of other residents a la Governor Andrew Cuomo. She also pushed lockdowns and masks, resulting in more deaths.

11. Monica Gandhi, M.D.

Absolutely wrong about lockdowns, masks and vaccines but with less of a platform than Drs. Wen and Walensky.

12. Celine Gounder, M.D.

Same as Monica Gandhi.

13. Erin Burnett

This CNN Host questioned Dr. Scott Atlas's qualifications for the job as advisor to President Trump. It was arguing from authority without having any. It was one of the most bizarre exchanges I have ever witnessed. Burnett was trying to tell Atlas that, because he used to be a neuro-radiologist, he wasn't qualified to advise on public health issues. Her little gambit came to an embarrassing end when he let her know about his 10 years researching Public Health Policy as a Fellow at the Hoover Institute.

14 Monica Ghandi, M.D.

Below the TV hostesses because they are repeating what she says and they have a much bigger platform. In a one-hour, fifteen minute podcast with Dr. Z (also known as Z-Dogg), she made the following claims:. 1. "

15. Katrine Wallace, PhD

(Please see Brianna Keilar, above)

9 *Best Trial Analysts*

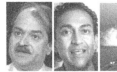

1. **John Ioannidis, M.D.**
2. **Vinay Prasad, M.D. MPH**
3. **JikkyLeaks**
4. **El Gato Malo**
5. **Alexandros Marinos**
6. **Jay Bhattacharya, M.D. PhD**
7. **Toby Rogers, PhD**
8. **Pierre Kory, M.D.**
9. **Peter McCullough, M.D.**

154 Who Received More Respect Than they Deserved

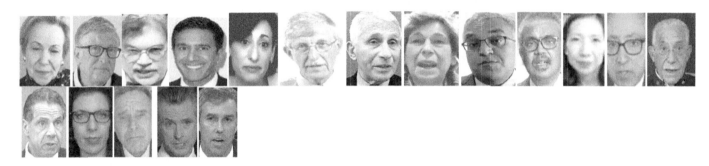

1. Deborah Birx

Dr. Birx and many others were wrong on lockdowns, the most destructive and deadly policy in the history of medicine. She is by far the worst offender because she helped institute and extend them by lying to Trump. She spelled it out clearly in her book. Then she violated the very mandate she forced on everyone else by flying to Delaware for a family gathering. Then she lied when asked about it. "It was immediate family", she said. (People were living in different houses). Don't let the scarves fool you. Such was the quality of the people running the show. Then she kept it out of her memoir as if it never happened.

She refused to talk to people invited to the White House for the purpose of discussing the harms and benefits of her policies even though group discussions of this kind are part of the job and the primary way public policy ideas get vetted. People were dying from these policies and they were not working as promised. Something needed to be done and her solution was to get out of town before the other experts arrived. It was a dereliction of duty of the highest order. I remember when she was introduced as part of the White House Advisory Team. Her colleagues talked about how competent and dedicated she was. She demonstrated herself to be neither of those. Read her memo to Mark Short below, dated 8.25.2020, entitled "I Just Can't"

I just can't.

From: "Birx, Deborah L. EOP/NSC" <███████████████████
Date: Tuesday, August 25, 2020 at 7:55 AM
To: "Short, Marc T. EOP/OVP" ███████████████████
Subject: FW: For Review: Draft POTUS Remarks - Meeting with Medical Experts

I can't be part of this with these people who believe in herd immunity and believe we are fine with only protecting the 1.5M Americans in LTCF and not the 80M + with co-morbidities in the populations included the unacceptable death toll among Native Americans, Hispanics and Blacks. With our current mitigation scenario we end up near 300K by Christmas and 500K by the time we have vaccine – close to the 600K live lost with 1918 Flu. We have worked to find a path that is the least disruptive to the economy but moves us under R1 and saves both the economy and American lives. Without masks and social distancing in public and homes we end up with twice as many deaths – we are a very unhealthy nation with a lot of obesity etc – we will never look as good as even Sweden due to our co-morbidities. These are people who believe that all the curves are predetermined and mitigation is irrelevant – they are a fringe group without grounding in epidemics, public health or on the ground common sense experience. I am happy to go out of town or whatever gives the WH cover for Weds. Perhaps do Annapolis and meet with Hogan. Fauci and I could probably do it together – I am open to options. Deb

Aside from refusing to meet with the experts invited to the White House, this memo proves she didn't understand respiratory virus transmission.

2. Bill Gates

I was surprised Bill let himself become so connected to Big Pharma and these horrible "vaccines". His big investment in BioNTech made in September of 2019 accounted for some of it but it was not a good move except from a business perspective. His lack of medical perspective for even the mathematical parts of medicine reflected very poorly on him. He was calling for tracing in October of 2020. That wouldn't have done any good in January, for a respiratory virus. Into 2021, he still thought SARS-2 entered the human population through natural zoonotic spillover and might still believe it. I don't know. If he *didn't* believe what he was saying, he was part of the cover-up, which is worse.
He said he and the doctors at the Gates Foundation hadn't realized the IFR was so low back in March of 2020. He wouldn't have known about my calculations but he and the doctors at the Gates Foundation should have known about Dr. Levitt's value of about .2%.
Finally, he was a staunch defender of Dr. Fauci's. Fauci was wrong on everything so, by extension, Gates takes on some of the idiotic policy endorsements, at least from a public relations perspective. He made a huge amount of money on the pandemic but he damaged his image profoundly.

3. Peter Hotez, M.D., PhD
4. Sanjay Gupta, M.D.
5. Rochelle Walensky, M.D.
6. Francis Collins, M.D., PhD
7. Anthony Fauci, M.D.
8. Randi Weingarten

Not knowing anything about medical science, while trying to influence the CDC on when schools should re-open means the motivation behind her actions had nothing to do with the well-being of children; not a good look for the President of a Teachers Union. The Democratic party purports to be on the side of underprivileged people. This was a slap in the face of children whose families could not afford tutors to keep them moving forward. They are more likely to drop out, will earn less, and will live shorter lives than those students whose families could afford private tutors, frequently the teachers from their schools who were on paid leave. Those teachers were getting two salaries.

9. Ashish Jha, M.D., MPH

He appears to not understand the medical science surrounding the pandemic, and gives the impression that he cannot interpret studies properly.

10. WHO DirectorTedros

11. Leana Wen, M.D.

12. Jonathan Reiner. M.D.

13. William Haseltine, PhD

14. Andrew Cuomo

15. Megan Ranney, M.D.

16. Eric Topol, M.D.

17. Eric Fiegl-Ding, PhD

18. Gavin Newsome

19. All other M.D.T.V. Mafia members

20. The former Stanford Medical School Dean, Philip A. Pizzo, M.D. and all 105 additional people who signed the letter denouncing Dr. Scott Atlas. (Please see a separate list for the names.)

21. The 27 scientists who signed the letter arranged by Peter Daszak, and published in the Lancet.

 Those people referred to the lab leak hypothesis as a conspiracy theory.

22. Beto O'Rourke

23. Avindra Nath, M.D.

Patients started reporting neurological injuries very early after receiving the vaccines. As Director of NINDS, the National Institute of Neurological Disorders and Stroke, Dr. Nath headed a team whose job it was to examine the neurologically-injured. There is some evidence that early on, he believed the injuries were linked to the vaccines. But a few months later, he changed his tune abruptly as neurological injuries accumulated. To this day, he refuses to acknowledge the clear link.

Tim Drug Hell's 9 Most Villainous Musicians

(non-bold comments by the author)

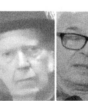

1. **Billy Bragg (Supports vax mandates for nurses.)**
2. **Bruce Springsteen (vax-only gigs)**

    Bruce, these vaccines do not prevent the transmission of virus from one person to another. Vax-only gigs make no sense and are probably counter-productive.
3. **Dave Grohl (Vax-only gigs.)**
4. **Dolly Parton for telling everyone to take the vax and reworking 'Jolene' as 'Vaccine, Vaccine.'**

    I don't think the business-savvy and kind-hearted Dolly would have done that if she had known about the almost worthless and terribly dangerous vaccines. But I can't give her a pass. It's her responsibility to find out before promoting something meant for public consumption.

5. **Kaiser Chiefs ("Hands up who's taken Moderna!")**
6. **Neil Young ("Take down Joe Rogan or I'm removing my music from Spotify.")**
   By trying to take Rogan down from interviewing people like Drs. Malone, McCullough, or me (I wish), Neil and Joni are supporting Big Pharma, The U.S. Government's nefarious activities during COVID, and Justin Trudeau and Theresa Tam from their native Canada, thereby becoming part of the corrupt establishment they once abhorred.
7. **Joni Mitchell ("Take down Joe Rogan or I'm removing my music from Spotify.")**
8. **UB40 for sacking singer Matt Hoy for not taking the vaccine**
9. **Tony Visconti for sacking (original Bowie drummer) Woody Woodmansey from Bowie tribute act Holy Holy for not taking vax even though he had a medical exemption**

106 *Stanford Medical School Physicians/Scientists Who Signed the Following Letter Denouncing Scott Atlas, M.D.*
(False statements and criticisms in bold)

September 9, 2020

Dear Colleagues,

As infectious diseases physicians and researchers, microbiologists and immunologists, epidemiologists and health policy leaders, we stand united in efforts to develop and promote science-based solutions that advance human health and prevent suffering from the coronavirus pandemic. In this pursuit, we share a commitment to a basic principle derived from the Hippocratic Oath: Primum Non Nocere (First, Do No Harm).To prevent harm to the public's health, we also have both a moral and an ethical responsibility to call attention to the falsehoods and misrepresentations of science recently fostered by Dr. Scott Atlas, a former Stanford Medical School colleague and current senior fellow at the Hoover Institute at Stanford University **[What falsehoods and misrepresentations of science are you referring to?]**. Many of his opinions and statements run counter to established science **[Which opinions?]** and, by doing so, undermine public-health authorities and the credible science that guides effective public health policy. The preponderance of data, accrued from around the world, currently supports each of the following statements:

• The use of face masks, social distancing, hand washing and hygiene have been shown to substantially reduce the spread of Covid-19. **[This is not supported by the data. Countries and States that employed these measures did not fare any better than neighboring countries and States that did. In addition, meta-analyses of randomized controlled trials did not show any significant reduction in transmission of respiratory viruses with the use of face masks and even hand-washing and hygiene.]** Crowded indoor spaces are settings that significantly increase the risk of community spread of SARS-CoV-2.

• Transmission of SARS-CoV-2 frequently occurs from asymptomatic people, including children and young adults, to family members and others. Therefore, testing asymptomatic individuals, especially those with probable Covid-19 exposure is important to break the chain of ongoing transmission. **[You can't break the chain of transmission of a respiratory virus spread by aerosols, by testing asymptomatic individuals. This was tried with the RT-PCR test and did not help. It was very** expensive and produced enormous numbers of false positives, distorting active case, hospitalization, and death counts.]

● Children of all ages can be infected with SARS-CoV-2. While infection is less common in children than in adults, serious short-term and long-term consequences of Covid-19 are increasingly described in children and young people.

● The pandemic will be controlled when a large proportion of a population has developed immunity (referred to as herd immunity) and that the safest path to herd immunity is through deployment of rigorously evaluated, effective vaccines that have been approved by regulatory agencies. **[We reached herd immunity to the Wuhan strain on January 11, 2021 without a single person having acquired the benefits of being fully-vaccinated. Of course, Dr. Pizzo and the other cosigners could not have known. The vaccines were neither rigorously evaluated nor effective nor were they all approved.]**

● In contrast, encouraging herd immunity through unchecked community transmission is not a safe public health strategy. **[I don't think Dr. Atlas encouraged herd immunity through unchecked community transmission.]** In fact, this approach would do the opposite, causing a significant increase in preventable cases, suffering and deaths, especially among vulnerable populations, such as older individuals and essential workers. Commitment to science-based decision-making is a fundamental obligation of public health policy. The rates of SARS-CoV-2 infection in the US, with consequent morbidity and mortality, are among the highest in the world. The policy response to this pandemic must reinforce the science, including that evidence-based prevention and the safe development, testing and delivery of efficacious therapies and preventive measures, including vaccines, represent the safest path forward. Failure to follow the science -- or deliberately misrepresenting the science – will lead to immense avoidable harm. We believe that social and economic activity can reopen safely, if we follow policies that are consistent with science. In fact, the countries that have reopened businesses and schools safely are those that have implemented the science-based strategies outlined above. **[Implementing mask use by the general public, social distancing, hand washing, and hygiene were not instrumental in safely reopening social and economic activity.]**

As Stanford faculty with expertise in infectious diseases, epidemiology and health policy, our signatures support this statement with the hope that our voices affirm scientific, medical and public health approaches that promote the safety of our communities and nation.

Dr. Pizzo: Your letter said nothing specific about Scott Atlas except implying that he "encouraged herd immunity through unchecked community transmission". I don't believe that was his position. The rest of the letter was either false or just fluff such as "The policy response to this pandemic must reinforce the science."
You wrote, "The use of face masks, social distancing, hand washing and hygiene have been shown to substantially reduce the spread of Covid-19". This is not true. See below. "Testing asymptomatic individuals, especially those with probable Covid-19 exposure is important to break the chain of ongoing transmission." This is also not true.
I am shocked that so many members of the faculty at the Stanford School of Medicine- many from the Department of Epidemiology- can't interpret data showing mask mandates did not reduce transmission significantly. I can understand why they might not understand mask science but all they had to do was a literature search if they didn't understand it or look at this year's data, which was plentiful at the time this letter was written. They also are endorsing asymptomatic testing with

the RT-PCR test. They clearly don't understand how that test works either. What good is testing asymptomatic people for a respiratory virus transmitted by aerosols? A positive result may come for months after a person has recovered because the test looks for viral fragments of nucleotides, not viable virus. Then they call it a new case when the test is positive, sometimes having used up to 40 cycles. Here are the results of 74 years of meta-analyses of randomized controlled trials showing masks do not reduce transmission significantly for respiratory viruses (influenza).

1. " Although mechanistic studies support the potential effect of hand hygiene or face masks, evidence from 14 randomized controlled trials of these measures did not support a substantial effect on transmission of laboratory-confirmed influenza." 2. "The evidence from RCTs suggested that the use of face masks either by infected persons or by uninfected persons does not have a substantial effect on influenza transmission". 3."In our systematic review, we identified 10 RCTs that reported estimates of the effectiveness of face masks in reducing laboratory-confirmed influenza virus infections in the community from literature published during 1946–July 27, 2018. In pooled analysis, we found no significant reduction in influenza transmission with the use of face masks." 4." The overall reduction in ILI or laboratory-confirmed influenza cases in the face mask group was not significant in either studies (9, 10)" From Emerging Infectious Diseases/NIH/U.S. National Library of Medicine https://www.ncbi.nlm.nih.gov/pmc/articles/PMC7181938/

Here are the people who signed the letter:

1. Philip A. Pizzo, M.D. and Professor of Pediatrics Former Dean, Stanford Sch. of Medicine
2. Upi Singh, MD Professor of Medicine and Chief Division of Infectious Diseases
3. Bonnie Maldonado, MD, Senior Associate Dean for Faculty Development and Diversity
4. Lucy Shapiro, PhD, Professor of Developmental Biology
5. Melissa Bondy, PhD, Professor and Chair of Epidemiology
6. Michele Barry, MD, Professor of Medicine
7. Charles Prober, MD, Professor of Pediatrics
8. Julie Parsonnet, MD, Professor of Epidemiology and Population Health
9. Steve Goodman, MD, MHS, PhD Professor of Epidemiology and Population Health
10. David Relman, MD, Professor of Medicine (Infectious Diseases)
11. Lee M. Sanders, MD, MPH Associate Professor of Pediatrics
12. Steve Luby, MD, Professor of Medicine, Epidemiology and Population   Health
13. Harry Greenberg, MD, Professor of Medicine and of
14. Ann Arvin, MD, Professor of Pediatrics (Infectious Diseases)
15. Edward S Mocarski Jr, PhD, Professor of Microbiology and Immunology
16. John Boothroyd, PhD, Professor of Microbiology and Immunology
17. John Carette, PhD, Assoc. Professor of Microbiology and Immunology
18. Dylan Dodd, MD, PhD, Assistant Professor of Pathology
19. Jason Andrews, MD, SM, Associate Professor of Epidemiology and Health Policy
20. David Studdert, LLB, MPH, ScD, Professor of Law and Medicine
21. Michelle Mello, JD, PhD, Professor of Medicine (Health Policy)
22. Joshua Salomon, PhD, Professor of Medicine (Primary Care)
23. Manuel Ricardo Amieva, , MD, PhD, Professor of Pediatrics
24. Lorene Nelson, PhD, MA, Associate Professor of Epidemiology
25. Abraham Verghese, MD, MACP, FRCP Professor
26. Aruna Subramanian, MD, Clinical Professor of Medicine

27. Dean L. Winslow, MD, FACP, FIDSA, FPIDS, Professor of Medicine
28. Stephen J Galli, MD, Professor of Pathology
29. Helen M Blau, PhD, Professor of Microbiology and Immunology
30. Jason Wang, MD, PhD, Associate Professor of Pediatrics and Medicine
31. Ann Hsing, PhD, MPH, Professor of Medicine and Epidemiology
32. Steve Asch, MD, MPH, Professor of Medicine, and Population Health
33. Esther John, PhD, MSPH, Professor, Department of Epidemiology
34. Thomas C Merigan, MD, Professor of Medicine
35. David A. Stevens, M.D., F.A.C.P., F.A.A.M., F.I.D.S.A., Prof. of Medicine
36. Gary K. Schoolnik, MD, Professor of Medicine -Infectious Diseases
37. Cornelia L. Dekker, MD, Professor of Pediatrics (Infectious Diseases)
38. Denise Monack, PhD, Professor of Microbiology and Immunology
39. Stan Deresinski, MD, FIDSA, Clinical Professor of Medicine
40. Shirit Einav, MD, Associate Professor Medicine- Infectious Diseases
41. Robert Shafer, MD, Professor of Medicine- Infectious Diseases
42. Holden Terry Maecker, PhD, Professor of Microbiology /Immunology
43. Wah Chiu, PhD, Professor of Bioengineering
44. Doug K Owens, MD, MS, Professor of Medicine
45. Cybele A. Renault, MD, DTM&H Clinical Associate Professor (ID)
46. Jake Scott, MD, Clinical Assistant Professor of Medicine
47. Justin Sonnenburg, PhD, Associate Professor of M&I
48. Hector Bonilla, MD, Clinical Associate Professor of Medicine (ID)
49. Dora Ho, MD, PhDClinical Associate Professor of Medicine (ID)
50. Marisa Holubar, MD MS, Clinical Associate Professor of Medicine
51. Sharon Chen, MD, MS, Clinical Associate Professor of Pediatrics (ID)
52. Roshni Matthew, MD, Clinical Assistant Professor of Pediatrics (ID)
53. Elizabeth S. Egan, MD, PhD, Assistant Professor of Pediatrics (ID)
54. Jenny R. Aronson, MD, Clinical Assistant Professor Division of ID
55. Catherine Blish, MD, PhD, Associate Professor of Medicine (ID)
56. Paul L. Bollyky, MD, D.Phil, Associate Professor Division of ID
57. Talal Seddick, MD, Clinical Assistant Professor of Pediatrics (ID)
58. Clea Sarnquist, MD, Clinical Professor of Pediatrics (ID)
59. Sruti Nadimpalli, MD, Clinical Professor of Pediatrics (ID)
60. Tim Stearns, PhD, Professor of Biology and of Genetics
61. Kerwyn Casey Huang, PhD, Professor of Bioengineering
62. Michael Fischbach, PhD, Associate Professor of Bioengineering
63. Maya Adam, MD, Clinical Assistant Professor of Pediatrics
64. Samantha Johnson, MD, MPH, Clinical Associate Professor of Pediatrics
65. Philip M. Grant, MD, Assistant Professor of Medicine (ID)
66. Joanna Nelson, MD, Clinical Assistant Professor Internal Medicine (ID)
67. A.C. Matin, PhD, Professor of Microbiology and Immunology
68. Taia T. Wang, MD, PhD, MSCI, Assistant Professor of Medicine
69. Peter Sarnow, PhD, Professor of Microbiology and Immunology
70. Hayley Gans, MD, Clinical Professor, Pediatrics -Infectious Diseases

71. Michael Baiocchi, PhD, Assistant Professor, Epidemiology
72. Glenn M. Chertow, MD, MPH, Professor of Medicine, and
73. Paul Graham Fisher, MD, Professor, Neurology and Pediatrics
74. Lisa Goldman-Rosas, PhD, MPH, Assistant Professor, Epidemiology
75. Bonnie Halpern-Felsher, PhD, FSAHM, Professor of Pediatrics
76. Victor Henderson, MD, Professor, Department of Epidemiology
77. Tina Hernandez-Boussard, PhD, MPH, MS, Assoc. Professor of Medicine
78. Abby King, PhD, Professor, Epidemiology and Population Health
79. Allison W. Kurian, M.D., M.Sc.Associate Professor of Medicine
80. Lianne Kurina, PhD, Associate Professor, PrimaryCare
81. Mitchell R. Lunn, MD, MAS, FACP, FASN, Assistant Prof. of Medicine
82. Kari Nadeau, MD, PhD, Professor of Pediatric Food Allergy, Immunology
83. Lorene Nelson, PhD, MSAssociate Professor, of Epidemiology
84. Mindie H. Nguyen, MD, MAS, AGAF, FAASLD, Professor of Medicine
85. Michelle C. Odden, PhD, Associate Professor, of Epidemiology
86. Juno Obedin-Maliver, MD, MPH, MAS, Assistant Professor of OB/GYN
87. Latha Palaniappan, MD, MS, FAHA, FACC, FACP Professor of Medicine
88. Lesley S. Park, PhD, MPH, Instructor, Department of Epidemiology
89. Rita A. Popat, PhD, Clinical Associate Professor, of Epidemiology
90. David H Rehkopf, ScD, MPH, Associate Professor of Epidemiology
91. Thomas N. Robinson, MD, MPH, Professor of Pediatrics
92. Kristin Sainani, PhD, Associate Professor of Epidemiology
93. Gary M. Shaw, DrPH, Professor of Pediatrics,
94. Julia F Simard, ScD, Associate Professor of Epidemiology
95. Marcia L. Stefanick, PhD, Professor of Medicine
96. Holly Tabor, PhD, Associate Professor, Department of Medicine
97. Alice S. Whittemore, Ph.D.Professor (Emerita) of Epidemiology
98. A. Desiree LaBeaud, MD, MS, Professor of Pediatrics (ID)
99. Robert Siegel, Professor (Teaching) of Microbiology and Immunology
100. Sara Singer, MBA PhD, Professor of Medicine Primary Care
101. David Schneider, PhD, Professor of Microbiology and Immunology
102. Matthew Bogyo, PhD, Professor of Pathology
103. Lucy S Tompkins, MD PhD, Professor of Medicine (ID)
104. Ami S. Bhatt, MD, PhD, Assistant Professor of Medicine
105. Anne Liu, MD, Clinical Associate Professor, Infectious Disease
106. David Katzenstein, MD, Professor of Medicine (emeritus)

1 Inaccurate Modeler

1. Neil Ferguson, PhD, Imperial College, London

In an attempt to estimate the number of deaths from Bird Flu in 2005, Dr. Ferguson stated that "Around 40 million people died in the 1918 Spanish flu outbreak. There are six times more people on the planet now so you could scale it up to around 200 million people probably".

74 persons, worldwide, died of Bird Flu in 2005. Estimates vary but less than 500 people died from Bird Flu over its entire course.

Professor Ferguson's past "worst-case" predictions vs. actual deaths			
	Mad cow disease	Swine flu	Bird flu
Prediction	150,000	65,000*	200,000,000
Actual	2,704	457*	455

* UK-only estimate
Sources: Lee Elliot Major, "BSE-infected sheep a 'greater risk' to humans," *The Guardian*, January 9, 2002; National CJD Research & Surveillance Unit, "Disease in the UK (By Calendar Year)," University of Edinburgh, May 4, 2020; Phillip W. Magness, "How Wrong Were the Models and Why?" American Institute for Economic Research, April 23, 2020; James Sturcke, "Bird flu pandemic 'could kill 150m,'" *The Guardian*, September 30, 2005; World Health Organization, "Cumulative Number of Confirmed Human Cases for Avian Influenza A(H5N1) reported to WHO, 2003-2020," January 20, 2020.

This time, he didn't do much better. Ferguson and his team at Imperial College, London, predicted that 81% of the population would become infected. They also assumed that the infection fatality rate for this virus was .9%. These two wildly-exaggerated figures lead to predictions of 600,000 people dying in the United Kingdom and 2.65 million dying in the U.S. And that's people actually dying because of (or "from") their COVID infection, i.e. not including "with" COVID. The total "because of" COVID probably hasn't reached 200,000 as of September 12, 2022 in the U.S. The over one million figure frequently quoted includes deaths "with" and "from". (Please see "8 Most Important Slides of the Pandemic")

In quoting 81% infected, he and his team appear to have overlooked a fact of exponential spread in a population. As the spread progresses, a larger and larger percentage of the population gets infected and either dies (in this case, about one person in 1000) or recovers from the disease and becomes immune. As this happens, smaller and smaller numbers of people are available to infect. This causes the R value to drop. To put this in perspective, consider that only 28% of the US population got infected during the 1918/1919 flu pandemic and only 22% in the 2009/2010 Swine flu epidemic.

The other error made by Dr. Ferguson's team was in not accounting for immunity-in place. At least 40% of the populations of England and the U.S. were protected from getting infected by the virus before it even arrived in the two countries. Real life examples of this phenomenon are nursing home patients who did not get the virus even though someone else in the nursing home did. The infected person would have exhaled virus into the poorly-ventilated space for weeks before he or she died. In such a case, the virus would have been floating around in all the rooms of the building. Why didn't all of the residents get infected? -because they had immunity-in-place. An earlier example comes from the cruise ship I used to calculate the correct IFR of .1%. Why did so many passengers on the Diamond Princess escape infection when an outbreak occurred there? -because they had immunity-in-place. Finally, to repeat, only about a quarter of the population got infected during the 1918/1919 Spanish

Flu and the 2009/2010 Swine Flu. Immunity-in-place greatly contributed to these surprisingly low numbers.

Dr. Ferguson's prediction of the percent infected at 81 was at least three times too high and possibly four. This scared politicians who don't understand this stuff and the result was idiotic policies like lockdowns, masks for the general population, school closures, etc., none of which did anything to slow the spread and in the cases of lockdowns and school closures, caused enormous damage, including death. A reasonable alternative explanation is that the powers that be understood it reasonably well and wanted to deploy these destructive policies so they could control the people, extract money from them by handing out enormous subsidies to the elite class, and make them dependent on the government for future exploitation. Making people dependent on the government is easily accomplished by taking away their jobs and giving out subsistence checks periodically. This prepares them for universal basic income.

All of this at very great cost in human suffering, paid for by innocent people. The WHO predicted 140 million would starve to death due to supply chain disruptions secondary to the lockdowns. Before COVID, we had finally gotten to the point where no one in the world starved (unless a warlord or someone restricted food for political reasons). Everyone in the world was getting enough food to survive. Now we are back at square two. Innocent children must bear the cost of having their schooling interrupted for one or two years in the form of lower living standards and shorter lives. All for someone's grand plan for the future.

23 M.D.s Who Got Major Parts of COVID-19 Terribly Wrong

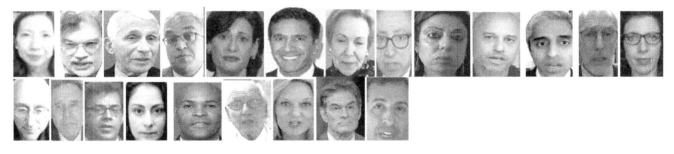

1. **Leana Wen, M.D**
2. **Peter Hotez, M.D., PhD**
3. **Anthony Fauci, M.D.**
4. **Ashish Jha, M.D., MPH**

Dr. Jha's bio includes seeing patients as an internal medicine clinician as well as his bureaucratic duties as Dean of the Brown University School of Public Health. Somewhere along the line, he became a go to TV commentator for all things COVID-19 on shows like Good Morning America and the major network Evening News broadcasts. Those venues require that you stick to the Narrative like glue even if you have to stray from the truth and Dr. Jha is a master at towing the line. This was noticed early on and explains why he was getting ten interview requests per day after only a few months removed from his first appearances. Most people know him as having recently been tapped by President Biden to take over as White House COVID-19 Response Coordinator and he has continued on the same track. That is, in fact, precisely why they brought him on. The White House can count on him to falsify trial results and lie about early treatment, if need be, to support very destructive policies such as vaccine mandates.

New on the job, he promptly stated, "There have not been any serious side effects of these vaccines." It's not likely that Dr. Jha has not heard about elevated risk of myocarditis in teenage boys with both the Pfizer and Moderna vaccines and clotting in young women with the Moderna vaccine. He is currently on a media tour promoting vaccines for six month to five-year-olds. He said, "It's really reassuring to know that for young kids, the vaccines are exceedingly safe." Saying that is not justified in any way. There is not a single trial that shows vaccines are safe for the six month to 5 years age group compared to the risk of bad outcomes from getting the disease. He said, "The vaccines are doing an extraordinary job at keeping kids out of the hospital". No, they're not. For Pfizer's vaccine the effectiveness at keeping kids out of the hospital is 22% after 60 days. That's a very poor showing, not "an extraordinary job".

Dr. Jha also said, "Ivermectin is great as a dewormer in horses. It does not work for COVID. We all wish it did. It doesn't. But thankfully we have drugs that do. Like Paxlovid. So if you get COVID — skip the Ivermectin and get a medicine that works." A word to the wise... If someone needs to say 'Ivermectin is a dewormer in horses', they are lacking in scientific evidence and have resorted to trying to besmirch the patient. Not a good look for a doctor... despicable, really.

Joe Rogan, the wildly successful podcaster, called Sanjay Gupta out on air for condoning everyone at CNN for saying in a very derogatory way, "Rogan took 'horse dewormer' when he got COVID." They did it every night for weeks. Rogan wasn't going to put up with that nonsense. As he once said, he has "fuck you" money. Finally, Gupta came on Rogan's show as a guest. Rogan confronted him with his behavior. Minutes went by as Dr. Gupta squirmed, but he couldn't wiggle his way out of it and finally admitted that CNN was out of line and as the medical guy over there, he was responsible for their demeaning of patients. Imagine a doctor you go to for help, looking the other way as people who are under his watch belittle patients on a daily basis. What kind of human being could do that even if he wasn't a doctor? The fact that he is, makes it that much more egregious.

When you thought Gupta could not possibly humiliate himself any further, he went on Don Lemon's show when he returned to the CNN building in Atlanta and changed his tune, participating in and endorsing others in the practice of demeaning those who are worried and sick and come to doctors for help in their time of need.

Drs. Jha and Gupta should know that most human medicines are used in animals. Ivermectin was developed for use in humans. It's used effectively for River Blindness in sub-Saharan Africa because it kills the parasite that causes loss of sight. People take it every week for prophylaxis. It's on the WHO essential medicines list. It was tried in COVID-19 when it worked spectacularly well in vitro against the SARS-2 virus. I wonder if Gupta and Jha would be man enough to go to sub-Saharan Africa and tell the people there that they are taking horse paste. They might not make it back to the US. When either or both of these doctor's mothers needs Coumadin, is he going to admit on television that she takes rat poison?
Stop this disgraceful demeaning of our fellow human beings in their time of need!
5. Rochelle Walensky, M.D.
6. Sanjay Gupta, M.D.
7. Deborah Birx, M.D.
8. Jonathan Reiner, M.D.
9. Monica Gandhi, M.D.
She thinks Japan had fewer cases of severe disease because they took up masks sooner than everyone else. So "blunt instrument", it's embarrassing. You think maybe their diet had something to do with it? Just to give you an idea of how wrong this person was and is, here are some quotes of hers from a

Zubin Damania, M.D. podcast: "The pandemic would have ended if the vaccines had been uptaken at a higher rate in the United States." She said this in September of 2021, nine months after I had shown that the vaccines did not prevent the virus from spreading. Listing countries who "were right about that (because they kept their uptake high, she started with the U'K who got their ass handed to them after their vaccine uptake was very high. The U.K. had more cases that almost every country including those who vaccinated the least. "As vaccines uptake has gotten better and better, society has become more and more open, even with Delta." Her big problem is that she confuses policy with what the virus is actually doing. She thinks society is becoming more open because vaccine uptake keeps going. Good lord. Statements like these from Dr. Ghandi go on for hours. In one podcast, she talks about studies showing that T cell immunity are mounted in response to (the viral) SARS-2 infection. If she didn't know this from medical school, she was asleep during immunology. She shouldn't have needed studies to know this. She thinks contact tracing works in September of 2021, more that a year and three quarters after the virus had been mixing throughout the population. Then she said "the B cell clonal memory cells that were made against the Wuhan strain will be directed against the variants". She said, "Three papers showed us that if the B cells produce antibodies, they will very cleverly be directed against the variants. That's how great our immune system is." Mondboggling...

10. Zubin Damania, M.D.

See above

He agrees with Dr. Ghandi constantly. They both still think vaccines work. Still thought in September 2021 that the unvaccinated were the ones in the hospital.

11. Vivek Murthy, M.D.

Dr. Murthy was the Surgeon General during a large part of the pandemic. I'm sure there was a lot of pressure on him from the administration to push the false narrative but that's no excuse. Lives were at stake and giving advice from the office of the Surgeon General of the United States of America is not kid stuff. I'm going to give him the benefit of the doubt and assume he was wrong because he didn't understand the medical science behind the SARS-2 virus, COVID-19 and the vaccines. I hope I'm right. It would be abhorrent to knowingly push a false narrative that clearly destroyed lives and caused the deaths of many innocent people.

Murthy was in favor of mandating vaccines for all employees of businesses of 100 or more of those employees. For someone to mandate an experimental injection when they, themselves, do not know the long term consequences, is just plain evil. I don't know how he could possibly not know this with all the resources at his disposal. In November of 2021, he said, "It's a necessary step to accelerate our pathway out of the pandemic." This quote shows that he was so out of it, he didn't even know that the vaccines did not prevent transmission of the virus, something I had proved 11 months earlier.

12. Gregory Poland, M.D.

The head of vaccinology at Mayo Clinic said in a podcast on September 1, 2022, "Because of the way we're handling this, there is yet another variant we're keeping our eye on. This will keep happening until, as a nation, we sort of come to the realization that a virus like this, as it has for the last 2 ½ years, is going to continue to mutate and continue to cause infections, long COVID and death until we're all immunized and until we're all wearing masks." This tells you all you need to know. He said "immunized" but he meant "vaccinated". If he meant "immunized", I'd want to know from him, exactly how someone can get immunized. The vaccine certainly won't do it. This doctor believes masks provide some kind of very significant amount of protection against getting infected such that if the entire nation began wearing them and got up to date on their vaccinations, the virus would stop mutating and there would never again be any infections, long COVID, or death.

13. Megan Ranney, M.D., MPH

14. Adam Cifu, M.D.

I wasn't familiar with this doctor's position until I saw a guest lecture and Q&A he did on Dr. Vinay Prasad's video channel. Here are two of his quotes from the video: "Reasonable people don't talk about using hydroxychloroquine or ivermectin." I don't think Dr. Cifu has looked at the trial results. And "Most of us would say, 'Vaccinate everybody'". Almost all age groups should not get this vaccine. You might be able to make a case for it in the oldest age groups.

Then I read a piece he wrote supporting vaccines in six- month-old babies to 11-year-olds. Here is a quote from that piece: 1. "Children, with and without comorbidities, should be vaccinated against COVID-19." Making a statement like this without considering how many children have already had the disease and thus have clonal memory makes no sense. When Dr. Cifu made this statement, the vaccine that was available was for the original Wuhan strain. No one knows the long-term side effect profile of this vaccine. In a disease where the risk of dying in young children is 1 in one million, you can't make a case for vaccinating all children 6 months to 11 years old

15. Eric Topol, M.D.

16. Atul Guwande, M.D.

Dr. Guwande only adopted two incorrect positions that I heard about but they were both egregious errors. One was in not endorsing a treatment that showed clear efficacy at a time when that efficacy had not been confirmed with a randomized, controlled trial or the equivalent. The other was in claiming that the immunity conferred by the vaccine which uses a viral subunit without an adjuvant- the weakest kind of vaccine- was superior to that conferred by getting and recovering from the disease; the strongest kind of immunity you can get because you get memory and clonal expansion for many antigens in and on the virus. Sad to say, but this demonstrates a profound lack of understanding of one of the most fundamental tenets of immunology

.

Why are the COVID vaccines so ineffective and short-lived?

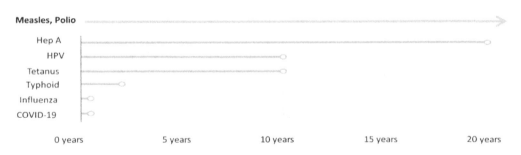

Tetanus is a component vaccine but has an adjuvant added, **COVID 19 's** only makes a component protein that changes its shape frequently. **Hep A's** killed vaccine protects for about 20 years.
The live attenuated vaccines of **measles and polio** protect far more than 99% of recipients for life.

17. Celine Gounder, M.D.

18. Jerome Adams, M.D.

19. Julie Parsonette, M.D.

20. Robert Redfield, M.D.

21. Tom Frieden, M.D.

22. William Schaffner, M.D.

A less prolific member of the M.D.T.V. Mafia (see below, Dr. Anne Rimoin)

23. Dr. Anne Rimoin, M.D.

See above

24. Mehmet Oz, M.D.

I've never understood Dr. Oz. He was a heart surgeon. I know a little about how hard it is to get to that level in the medical world. What I don't know is why he would throw it all away to do his TV show. It couldn't be for the money. It seems like a huge step down to me. Now he's running against a person who has no business being a Senator. He'd better win... He has been wrong on most things, COVID-19, including school closures, masks, vaccines, etc. Just clueless.

25. Roger Sheheult, M.D.

Still doesn't know the correct IFR on October 17, 2022. Been wrong on a number of things. Like Vinay Prasad, M.D. and John Campbell, PhD, he suffers from being "Trial bound" (relies on trials at the expense of thinking.)

7 Most Blatant Revisionist Historians

The lowest of the low. It's when you take the wrong stance on an issue and later claim that you were on the right side the whole time.

1. **Anthony Fauci, M.D.**

   Now claims he didn't endorse lockdowns. Now claims he was always open to both natural zoonotic spillover and the lab leak theory. The truth is that he called people conspiracy theorists who presented evidence it was modified or made from scratch in a lab. It is worth noting one major mistake Fauci made on which he hasn't changed his stance. He still thinks school closures were a good idea. When the example of Sweden showed the children and teachers were not at risk, Fauci pushed to keep schools closed "at least until the adult vaccines come out". When that happened, and the teachers had gotten vaccinated, Fauci was still against opening schools . He still tries to justify school closures, even to this day.

2. **Deborah Birx, M.D.**

   Now claims she knew the vaccines wouldn't block transmission before they came out on December 14, 2020. This is contradicted by a statement she made at the time.

3. **Peter Hotez, M.D., PhD**

   Now claims he was against school closings.

4. **Bill Gates**

   Now claims he and the doctors at the Gates Foundation didn't know the IFR was very low, roughly equal to the seasonal flu.

   Dr. Levitt and I, independently, calculated the infection fatality rate to be .1% (me) and around .2% (Dr. Levitt). I apologize for not being able to find the exact number for Dr. Levitt. Our results are not identical because we made different assumptions about for example, the steepness of the age distribution, the health differences between the average 80 year-old at home and an 80 year-old who is out on the high seas. We had our results by March 8. Other people tried to calculate this in late March or April. Their results were too high, ranging from 1% to about 2% depending on how many of the people they assigned to COVID who died several weeks later at home. Those people didn't take into consideration the fact that the average number of days from onset to death in COVID was 18.

I don't think Gates is being honest here about he and his team not knowing the IFR was very low. The WHO, CDC, China Medical, Italy, Germany, etc. had it too high at about 4% average. This was of the initial lies that threw the public into a state of fear enough to scare them into lockdowns. Bill also claims that he and Foundation docs didn't know it was a disease of the very old. Update: Bill wrote an article that was published in the New England Journal of Medicine, dated February 18, 2020 that verifies he and his B&MGF doctors knew the IFR was low and that it was a disease of the elderly. (please see #9 of "**9 *Most Important Slides of the Pandemic***" in Chapter 3). It confirms Bill's dishonesty lately regarding the time he learned the IFR was very low and that it was a disease of the elderly. He knew it was lower than the "experts" were saying, just not how low.

5.   **Peter Daszak, PhD**
     Now claims he didn't do some of the things that are spelled out in a tweet of his, dated November 21, 2019

6.   **Francis Collins, M.D., PhD**

7.   **Monica Ghandi, M.D.**

4 *Who Argued From Authority Most Disgracefully*

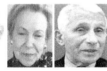

1. Jerome Adams, M.D.

A very alert woman from Georgia noticed a mistake made by the CDC in their ranking of causes of death in the pediatric age group. This doctor said something like (paraphrasing) "leave the scientific work to the qualified people." But she was right. He was wrong. Then he said. This conversation is over"- or something like that. It was shameful

2.Francis Collins, M.D., PhD

3. Deborah Birx, M.D.

Refusing to meet other doctors is arguing from authority. She wouldn't meet three other doctors who came to the White House to discuss lockdown policy. She thought they were out of line in their thinking. They had some good ideas it turns out. She was wrong in her assessment and clearly does not understand the science underlying SARS-2 and COVID-19.

4. Anthony Fauci, M.D.

Dr. Fauci once said he was "the Science". He has very little science background, as it turns out. He majored in The Classics in college at Holy Cross. He hasn't taken care of patients in quite a while.\

5. Marty Makary, M.D.

On June 15, 2020 Dr. Makary said, " ... and we can have those debates (of mask effectiveness). We have a country of opinions and we need to put those opinions aside. Whatever the effectiveness of the mask is, whether it's a 30% mitigation or a 60% mitigation in reducing the velocity of transmission, it's one of the few tools we have. Look at Asia, look at Europe. Look at many of the states in the northern United States. They have been able to manage the infection after initial spikes and surges because of universal masking."

All of this is wrong but what puts him on this list is that he talks about putting other peoples' opinions to the side. No, you can't do that. You're saying that because you're a docto0r and they aren't, their opinions should be put to the side. You have to win the argument with logic, not your degree. Clearly, you didn't understand the science of respiratory transmission of a virus 100 nm in diameter. Would you say to a layman, listen to you because you know how a gall bladder should be removed because you are a surgeon? No you would cut their argument to shreds with logic (I hope).

9 Blatant Flip-Floppers

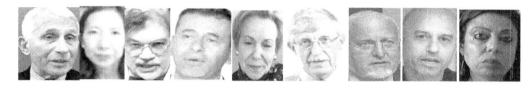

Flip-flopping happens when either, 1) more data comes in that makes someone want to change their position on an issue or policy, 2) political winds change, or 3) they change to be in the majority without regard to the data.

Flip-flopping is not the same as being a revisionist historian, its more dishonest cousin. Someone who was in favor of lockdowns, mask mandates, or school closures who now lies and says they were always in the right camp is a revisionist historian.

You would think this is done only by people who have never written anything or been in a recorded interview because it would be too easy to prove that they are lying when they say they have been on the right side the whole time. But people like Drs. Fauci and Birx, don't seem to mind if there is evidence out there that proves they are lying. Believe it or not, these two and others such as Dr. Peter Hotez will try to rewrite history by saying they were on the right side all along. Then someone comes along with proof of what they were preaching several months earlier. They don't seem to care. No shame.

In truth, there were very few, if any, people who were against any of these destructive policies in the beginning. Those few would have been the very rare who think in principles, and even more rare, those who reason from first principles. These are the most fundamental principles that apply to a problem and they do not change. Thus, those who reason using them do not change their minds mid-stream. They will either tell you they aren't sure about something or they will be able to say, "It's this way and here is why."

The plurality of flip-floppers are those who change their minds on an issue when they see that almost everyone else has changed theirs. They don't scrutinize the data very carefully. They go with the most popular narrative, flavored with irrelevant things like political leanings, social pressures, threats of losing their licenses to practice medicine, etc. and latch on to any explanation they hear that is consistent with the position held by most people. These are the sheep we hear about all the time.

Related but not exactly the same are those who change with the political winds. Leana Wen is a perfect example. She pushed lockdowns for about two years in accordance with her far-left political ideology. When it became too politically-damaging to continue, she turned against lockdowns. After all those people starved to death due to supply chain disruptions, she now calls lockdowns a "non-starter."

The third most common are the flip floppers who make their proclamations based on the data as it comes in or if they get convinced by someone who really understands the issue. There's nothing wrong with this as long as they don't try to rewrite history. Data, as you know by now, can be very difficult to interpret correctly. These flip-floppers misinterpret the data and make incorrect claims. Inevitably, someone comes along who correctly interprets that same data and takes the opposite position. More and more data comes in and it becomes overwhelming. The flip-flopper then changes his stance on an issue. They don't think in principles or they would not have made the mistake in the first place.

Here are 7 Flip-Floppers of the Last Two-and-a-Half Years.

1. Anthony Fauci, M.D.

Dr. Fauci is both a flip-flopper and a revisionist historian. He's a flip-flopper on masks and a revisionist historian on his willingness to be open minded about the origins of the virus.

I don't know whether Dr. Fauci would admit that he used to be a proponent of natural immunity because the entire year, he discounted it saying if you got the disease and recovered, you still need to get the vaccine. If he won't admit that he lied to the public all of 2020 and into 2021, ask him about the video located here: https://www.youtube.com/watch?v=Y_MeeYbYtWc

In another example, Dr. Fauci famously said in an early March, 2020 interview that he didn't see any reason why people should be going around wearing masks. Then, without anything changing, he was recommending masks. Privately, he was telling friends in emails, that they didn't need to wear masks. By October, he was recommending two masks. Also in October of 2020, at his alma mater, College of the Holy Cross, he said, "When it became clear that we had community spread in the country ... I recommended to the president that we shut the country down". He now claims he never recommended lockdowns.

As a fourth example, consider Dr. Fauci's position early on; that the virus could not have arisen from a lab. He went to great lengths to direct the Proximal Origins paper written the same day as the infamous teleconference arranged by Fauci and Jeremy Farrar. The paper was signed by five scientists, three of whom got increases in their funding for the next year. He also went around calling people conspiracy theorists who brought up the fact that all the evidence pointed to a lab origin of the virus. Fauci now says he always had an open mind about the origins of the virus. No, Dr. Fauci you actively engaged in attacking the character of people who spoke up about the origin being from a lab.

This is the common m.o. used by perpetrators. At first, when the issue is hot and the punishment for lying would be severe, they stick to their guns, even fabricating evidence and papers (in this case) to exonerate themselves. Later, when things have cooled somewhat and time has revealed the fabrications, they claim that they were always open to either interpretation. I say No! Calling people with opposing views "conspiracy theorists", especially when they are correct, is not being open to either interpretation. There are tons of examples of Fauci and Francis Collins doing this.

2. Leana Wen, M.D.

She used to be one of the world's biggest proponents of lockdowns.. For two years, on almost a daily basis, she pushed for deadly lockdowns. Then she turned against lockdowns. Nothing changed, except for the political winds, and she was against them. She still needs to be put on trial for her share of all the people who will die from from lockdowns (140 million will starve to death according to the WHO plus those dying now because of the moratorium placed on all but emergency surgery). She should be sent to prison if found guilty. As it stands now, she's going to walk away scot free and, most likely, do the same thing next time. As far as I can tell, she hasn't flipped away from masks and vaccine mandates. Yet.

Update: Summer of 2022 "For those who don't agree that the vaccinated can return to pre-pandemic normal, I ask: What should we all do? Perpetual masking? Forever not dining out, avoiding large weddings & indoor gatherings, etc.? Virtually everything has risk, and zero covid is not a viable strategy." -Leana Wen

3. Peter Hotez, M.D.

He claimed in a tweet that he was against school closures all along. I had just seen this quote of his embedded in an absurd take of his as to why the mismanagement (in his eyes) of the pandemic by Trump "threatened our homeland security". In this interview, he said, "Teachers will be terrified, and appropriately so, about going back to work." That's not being against school closures. He's an example of someone who lets his political ideology dominate his medical reasoning and reasoning in general. This interview was all about instilling fear in the public and trying to make Trump look bad before the elections of 2020. "..we will reach a point where people feel scared about going outside. And that's when homeland security is threatened. So this has to be recognized as a direct threat to our homeland security. And, right now, unfortunately, the way the White House is conducting its business, it's guaranteeing that our homeland security will be threatened." He used the phrase "threat to our homeland security" or "homeland security threatened" three times in three sentences. All for a virus that caused 2.6% of 1% of 1% per 100,000 people per month over the average of 2015 – 2019. It was fear-mongering and political attacks over something that was tiny, without regard to the damage he was doing to all but the richest school-age children. (please see #7 of 10 *Most Important Slides of the Pandemic*.")

4. Marty Makary, M.D.

Dr. Makary was in favor of lockdowns and mask use by the general public at first. Here's a quote of his from June 15, 2020: "… and we can have those debates (of mask effectiveness). We have a country of opinions and we need to put those opinions aside. Whatever the effectiveness of the mask is, whether it's a 30% mitigation or a 60% mitigation in reducing the velocity of transmission, it's one of the few tools we have. Look at Asia, look at Europe. Look at many of the states in the northern United States. They have been able to manage the infection after initial spikes and surges because of universal masking." This is so shocking. Masks provide close to zero % mitigation, to use his units. He's talking about 30% - 60%. It's a good thing he has flipped on this issue but he should have read the literature beforehand. On top of this, Dr. Makary is a surgeon. He uses surgical masks every day in the O.R. He should have known we use masks as "splash guards". They don't block anything as small as a 100 nanometer virus particle going in or out. My rebuttal to Dr. Makary's comment can be seen in "20 Stupid Quotes Surrounding the Pandemic".

5. Deborah Birx

With Dr. Birx, it's mostly revisionist history. She said "I knew these vaccines were not going to protect against infection." If she really knew this, why didn't she speak up? I didn't think they would protect against infection either and I made videos explaining it. I proved my suspicions correct in mid-January, less than a month after administration started and posted a video about it, on YouTube. But I was getting shadow-banned by YouTube. Birx had a huge platform. She could have told the world. I'd like to know how she proved she was correct. I don't think she is capable of the kind of analysis I used, for one because she hadn't acknowledged immunity-in-place which was critical to my proof.. Update: She wasn't telling the truth. I have uncovered a quote from around the same time (December 15, 2020, the day before the vaccines were released) that clearly implies she thought the vaccines would protect against infection. "To truly achieve herd immunity, it's going to take through the summer and potentially even into the fall," she said. "That's getting 70-80% of Americans immunized." If the vaccines don't block transmission, they don't do anything to help us reach herd immunity. So Dr. Birx is not telling the truth when she said recently, "I knew these vaccines were not going to protect against infection."

6. Francis Collins

Dr. Collins called people who advanced the lab origin of the virus, "conspiracy theorists". You won't hear him say that now that the evidence is overwhelming. He also said "Masks prevent the spread of COVID" (on video, no less). I hope he has enough sense to refrain from saying that now.

7. Robert Redfield

The former CDC Director flip-flopped on the origin of SARS-2. Again, it's ok to do this if you admit you were wrong, but there was plenty of evidence as soon as the genome was shared (and you didn't need the genome to prove it came from a lab. He also was completely wrong about the efficacy of masks, saying in testimony once that "this mask" (a surgical mask) protected him "better than a vaccine that is 70% effective." In fairness to him, this was before these vaccines came out. Assuming he meant traditional vaccines, he's very wrong and doesn't say this anymore. Masks don't reduce transmission significantly and never have. Look at the studies, doctor.

8. Zubin Damania, M.D.

Going with the popular opinion at the beginning (or maybe hedidn't understand the medical science and reasoned things out incorrectly (like most people)) really hurt Dr. Z-dogg; agreeing with Monica Ghandi in a few interviews finished him off. He's similar to Marty Makary; completely wrong on most things at the beginning, they backpedaled vigorously.

9. Monica Ghandi, M.D.

Wrong about almost everything at first. Tried unsuccessfully tochange her tune on masks buton September of 2022, said cloth masks because they kept a humid environment in people's mouthe and this reduced severe disease. Look at the data please, doctor.

8 TV "Experts" to Whom the Public Looked for Explanations Who Were Wrong on Virtually Every One of the Following Major calls (Mask Use by the General Public, Lockdowns, School Closures, Testing and Tracing, the Need for a Large Percentage of the Population to be Vaccinated Before We Could Reach Herd Immunity, Vaccine Efficacy, Whether or Not the Vaccines Could Block Transmission, Vaccine Safety, etc.)

The cumulative deaths caused by this group is over 100 million innocent souls many of them small children who have and will starve to death because of the supply chain disruptions secondary to the lockdowns.

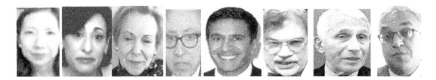

1. Leana Wen, M. D.
1. Rochelle Walensky, M.D.
1. Deborah Birx, M.D.
1. Jonathan Reiner, M.D.
1. Sanjay Gupta, M.D.
1. Peter Hotez, M.D., PhD
1. Anthony Fauci, M.D.
1. Ashish Jha, M.D. MPH

10 Scientists Up to Their Necks in the Cover-up of the SARS-2 Lab Origin

1. Peter Daszak, PhD

Daszak lied about there being live bats in the Wuhan Lab. He wrote his own "alibi" letter regarding the origin of the virus- calling it a conspiracy theory- and got 26 scientists to sign it. Then he got it published in the Lancet. The 2018 DARPA Proposal. The 2019 Tweet. Why the Senators and Congressmen don't subpoena this person to appear as an under oath witness in a congressional hearing is beyond comprehension.

2. Francis Collins, M.D., PhD

Dr. Collins is on record in numerous instances, referring to the Lab Leak Hypothesis as a "conspiracy theory," for months after I had proved this theory to be correct. The best reasons I can come up with for this truly bizarre position is that 1) the NIH, during the time Collins was director, supplied funding for the gain of function research that took place in China, so any incompetence by a lab subcontracted for this purpose would reflect poorly on the NIH and clearly demonstrate that the virus that is believed to have killed 6 million people worldwide was funded by the NIH with Collins as Director, 2) that Investigations of a lab leak would open a can of worms that would lead back to the corruption in that organization that has come to light recently (the $350 million in paybacks to NIH and NIAID employees) and 3) reveal that the royalties generated by the Moderna vaccine were shared with the NIH, with NIH-funded Daszak performing some of the reckless field research used by Moderna in the development of their vaccine. Or there could be other reasons.

3. Anthony Fauci, M.D.

4. Shi Zheng li

When Dr. Shi claimed in a Scientific American interview that the six miners who got infected in the Mojiang bat caves got fungal pneumonia when the radiological evidence clearly showed viral pneumonia, Could she have been covering up evidence of a connection between this incident and the spread of SARS-2 from the lab. Then Dr. Shi removed the viral genome sequences from the WIV website, possibly at the urging from someone at the NIH or the Galveston National Lab. She said it was because it was getting too many hits but if that was the case, she could have put it somewhere, password-protected, so people would still have access to it. Could she have done it to keep people from finding the precursor to SARS-2?

5. Kristian Andersen, PhD

Lead author of "The Proximal Origin of SARS-CoV-2", the paper written the day after the late-night group phone call arranged by Jeremy Farrar for Anthony Fauci. See "8 Disturbing Emails"

6. Ian Lipkin

"Proximal Origin" co-author with 5, 8, 9, and 10

7. Robert Garry, PhD

8. Edward C. Holmes, PhD

9. Andrew Rambaut, PhD

10. James Le Duc, PhD

The Director of the Galveston National Labs where many of the Chinese scientists trained in bio-safety protocols and virological procedures, he stayed close to the Narrative throughout and downplayed the lab origin theory.

1,000,000 Physicians/Scientists Most Cowardly in Refusing to Stand Up and Expose the Fraud and Deception When They Knew Better

"Were the people evil or just stupid who endorsed lockdowns, masks, school closures, vaccine mandates in general, vaccines for people who had already had the disease, vaccines in children based on those pathetic trials, etc.,?" I get asked this question almost every day. I would add one more category, that of "cowardly".

The cowards are the ones who knew bad information was coming out of their respective institutions but were afraid to speak up due to fear of losing their status, position, or income. These people put money ahead of other people's lives, particularly children's lives. Private doctors- the fellow or lady down the street who knew nonsense was coming from the CDC, or knew the trials the FDA used to approve vaccines in small children did not justify approval, etc. and didn't speak up in a timely fashion, were also cowards.

It sounds harsh to say it this way but anyone who would put their bank account before the lives of children needs some harsh talking to. This includes ANYONE who now says they knew all along that the vaccines were dangerous. They are cowards for not speaking up. The first thing you as a reader of this book should ask people who say "I knew lockdowns and masks wouldn't work" (trying to be smart, but of course no one really knew save for that one guy who was overseas and had proved they couldn't work- hell, even Scott Atlas has admitted that he thought at the time, lockdowns were worth a try- no, I'm talking about the guy who's trying to rewrite history to look smart- that guy has to answer, "If that's true, why were you too cowardly to say something about it?" Having to keep their job to take care of their family is not an excuse when people are dying in the tens of millions. Selling your Mercedes and driving a Toyota for two years will take care of your family just fine. And that's if you can't find another job WHICH NEVER HAPPENS TO DOCTORS. I call B.S. on the doctors who say they couldn't speak up for fear of losing their jobs while millions of children were starving to death due to supply chain disruptions secondary to lockdowns. Oh Boo Hoo, they're going to have to find another job or drive a Toyota for a year. Good Lord people, stop making excuses for multi-millionaire doctors losing a few dollars. If they really understood what was being done to humankind and didn't speak up about it, they are cowards or they put the comfort of driving around in a Mercedes, or just their bank account, ahead of the lives of other human beings starving to death. That's selfishness to the point of evil. I'd rather be dumb than cowardly or evil. Nothing is worse than a man who tries to cover his pathetic ass by saying his "hands were tied" career-wise (which is really just financially) so he couldn't speak up. Almost nothing disgusts me more about this whole thing than hearing this now. The truth is, all of this death and destruction would never have happened if the medical profession as a whole and every single doctor in it who knew people were being taken advantage of, had stood up and taken a stand for their fellow man, woman, and child. If you feel yourself trying to come up with an excuse for not doing what you could by speaking out against the evildoers, put a lid on it and admit you were wrong to have kept silent. That way, you can hope to salvage the little bit of dignity you have left. And try to do better next time.

The answer to the question posed at the beginning of this heading, about the people who went along when they knew better- were they evil or just stupid- is: neither. They were cowards. I hope this book will help you understand which of the three, stupid, evil, or coward- applies in different cases.

1. Physician/Scientist employees of major medical institutions all around the world who did not speak up when they realized evil was being perpetrated on innocent citizens including children as young as six months of age.

Some doctors and scientists have become increasingly aware that the information and authorizations released by the major medical institutions is frequently false and very damaging. They are trying to make excuses for putting money and career before the lives of children as young as six months of age. Everyone working at the CDC, FDA, NIH, NIAID and analogous institutions in countries throughout the world are either stupid, evil, or cowards. If they recognized the trial results to be inadequate to make several of the recommendations they have made for boosters, vaccine administration in children, etc., and did not speak up for fear of losing money or having their career disrupted, they are cowards who put money ahead of the lives of children. If they did not realize the recommendations were unwarranted, they are stupid. If they recognized it and signed off on them anyway, they are evil. There's really no other option.

Here are some quotes from the cowards who knew the public was being taken advantage of, including baby children who, at six months of age, were not yet old enough to be able to walk or talk :

"There's a silence, an unwillingness for agency scientists to say anything. Even though they know that some of what's being said out of the agency is absurd." – an NIH Scientist. Speak up next time! Look at the shape we're in now because of people like you who wouldn't speak up!.

"It's like a horror movie I'm being forced to watch and I can't close my eyes," one senior FDA official lamented. "People are getting bad advice and we can't say anything."

Really Mr. Senior FDA official, you "can't say anything"? Man up or woman up, whatever you are, and SPEAK UP. People died and will still die because of what you kept quiet about, especially small children and babies.

2. Andrew Hill Watch this video: https://www.oraclefilms.com/alettertoandrewhill

3. Ordinary medical doctors working in Universities and private practice who knew the science was being misrepresented and people were getting abused but refused to speak up. I've heard it said that doctors didn't have time to follow what was happening. This is a pathetic excuse. What medical doctor doesn't know that getting and recovering from a disease confers better protection than a subunit vaccine? Yet very few people stood up and said, "No, You're wrong", when Dr. Fauci, Atul Gawande and others claimed the vaccines conferred better immunity than that which you gain from recovering from the disease.

23 Men Responsible for the Most Death and Destruction

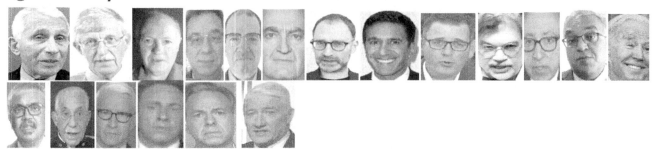

1. Anthony Fauci, M.D.

Dr. Fauci was involved in every aspect of this, from laying the groundwork for the virus to be created, to endorsing lockdowns, mask use by the general public, and school closures all the way to pushing the public into taking a vaccine with clear safety issues and marginal efficacy in only a small subgroup of patients even if they'd had the disease and recovered from it.

And before all that, he was instrumental in getting around the moratoria placed on gain of function research by moving it overseas to the labs of one of our archenemies.

Everything Dr. Fauci did, made the situation worse. He increased suffering and the loss of lives and cost America trillions of dollars. Lockdowns, delayed treatment causing people to get needlessly sick, school closures, small business closures, increased morbidity and mortality in future years arising out of the moratorium placed on all but emergency surgery, etc. You name it, he was behind it

2. Francis Collins, M.D., PhD

The NIH Director turned the proceedings into a circus by calling people conspiracy theorists when they knew more than he knew about the science surrounding COVID-19 or when they got a little too close to the truth about his involvement in the creation of the SARS-2 virus. That's why he is ranked second on this list. He was right there at the beginning, funding Eco-Health Alliance which subcontracted out some of the work to the Wuhan Institute of Virology where the vaccine was created.

His reputation was further tarnished by the scandal involving payments from Big Pharma back to NIH employees including to him and NIH's refusal to disclose the information until taken to court and forced by a judge. Even after the judge's order, the NIH is slow walking the release and the documents are heavily redacted.

Someone with the stature of Dr. Collins should never have risked his place in history in this way. He led the U.S. part of the Human Genome Project which began in 1990 and was completed in 2003 and was one of the top five milestones achieved in the biological sciences in the 20th Century. All Dr. Collins had to do was admit to a few errors of judgment regarding his funding of projects in China and stay above the fray. He would have skated through, at least until the kickback scandal erupted.

3.Peter Daszak, PhD

Dr. Daszak was the man on the ground doing the reckless research with bats in the Yunnan, China caves. (Please see "3 Reasons We Can Be Sure There Was Planning Beforehand")

4. Neil Ferguson, PhD

Ferguson grossly overestimated the number of deaths from the pandemic, instilling fear. He then pushed for lockdowns which was the exact opposite of what needed to be done.

5. Albert Bourla, DVM

Think for a second about the influence of companies like Pfizer (and a few others) on your lives and those you love. Entire networks could not exist without them, networks that promote treatments approved by governmental regulating bodies without regard to whether those treatments are worthless or even dangerous or outright harmful, based on trial results paid for and in many cases manipulated, by those same companies. This means that people, in whom the public places the health of their children, must tow the company line or they are out the door. This includes lying about the efficacy and safety of a product, if necessary.

The networks have to hire the type of people who place their bank accounts above the lives of six-month-old children for this to work and Albert Bourla is at the top of it all when it comes to Pfizer. Here's how it works: Albert Bourla approves advertising dollars to be put toward CNN programming, without which they could not exist. CNN hires a lot of people of low enough integrity that they are willing to gin up fear of a virus that has an infection fatality rate about equal to seasonal influenza. Those show hosts (John Berman, Brianna Keilar, Alisyn Camerota, Chris Cuomo, Poppy Harlow, Don Lemon, Anderson Cooper, Erin Burnett, etc.) push the fear narrative, and besmirch and censor doctors who can show the narrative is misleading and harmful. All of this is done relentlessly, setting the stage for their doctor, Sanjay Gupta, M.D. to get on that enormous platform and spew utter nonsense with a smile on his face, harmful nonsense, nonsense about a medical phenomenon too complicated for the public to understand such that they put their faith in his wisdom regarding how to avoid getting infected, and how to treat it if they do.

Gupta was active in pushing the false narrative from the very beginning, including the absurdly too-high infection fatality rate, and the harmful policies that went along with it, including mask use by the general public- even cloth masks-, lockdowns, school closures, etc. In fairness, Dr. Gupta probably was part of the 99.999999 %- of the US population that thought these interventions might help as there was only one of us who could prove they couldn't help at that time, furthermore that they would set us on a path of colossal destruction for years to come.

With the ultimate goal of subsuming private and public monies into the coffers of Pfizer for a vaccine that was turning out to be unsafe let alone ineffective in ongoing trials, Supreme Commander Bourla knew how important his Propaganda Division would continue to be and considered Field Marshal Gupta far more valuable than the utterly-replaceable General Jeff Zucker. "Gupta", he reminded himself, many times through the summer and early fall, "was more important than BioNTech, the whole lot of them, because it didn't matter so much what they were injecting into arms as it was getting those arms to line up and be scared enough to want it or at least think they needed it."

The other Divisions Bourla had to manage were Censorship, Government, and Medical Science. He was also involved in the CCP through Fosun ending up manufacturing Pfizer vaccines in Boston, MA and Princeton, NJ

6. Stephane Bancel

7. Moncef Slaoui, PhD

How could Trump have hired someone to head Operation Warp Speed with so many conflicts of interest in the Pharmaceutical Industry? Without question, the worst hire of his Presidency except for Omarosa Manigault Newman, this guy had been retired for three years. He was working as a Board member at Moderna among others and as a consultant to several Big Pharma companies while retaining substantial stock holdings in many of them. Was he such an incredibly talented leader and effective businessman that Trump couldn't find someone else to take on what could reasonably be considered the most important job to date of the new millennium? No, he wasn't. As Head of R&D at Glaxo Smith Kline, he spearheaded three major deals, all of which were dismal failures. One veteran pharmaceutical executive called them, "three of the worst deals in drug industry history."

8. Neil Ferguson, PhD

Ferguson grossly overestimated the number of deaths from the pandemic, instilling fear. He then pushed for lockdowns which was the exact opposite of what needed to be done.

9. Sanjay Gupta, M.D.

Having an enormous platform comes with the responsibility to refrain from misleading the public yet Dr. Gupta did this on a daily basis. Like the rest of the "M.D.T.V. Mafia", he was wrong on virtually every call. When he wasn't showing people how to wash their hands or wipe down their groceries, he was distributing homemade facemasks that gave people a sense of false protection. He also allowed Alyson Camerota to make bizarrely illogical statements on air without correcting her and reinforced the incorrect IFR months after I and others had proved that the experts had it 40x too high.

And what about the way he conducted himself in supporting the notion that people who were taking ivermectin, were taking "horse paste" when every doctor knows ivermectin is a very safe drug that was developed for humans, and has shown efficacy against a large handful of viruses since 2012. He was publically humiliated by Joe Rogan on Rogan's podcast for refusing to agree that it was improper for the CNN hosts to say, "Joe Rogan is taking horse paste." Gupta resisted but Rogan was having nothing of it and Gupta finally relented and admitted it was wrong for CNN to have done that. Then Gupta appeared on Don Lemon's show a few days later and went back on what he had acknowledged on Rogan's show. Gupta's reputation suffered tremendously from the way he handled the horse paste issue and he deserved it. But being incorrect on virtually everything involving the science behind COVID-19 is what damaged his reputation the most. He was showing people how to wash their hands and told the viewers his family wiped down their groceries for a respiratory virus that is transmitted by aerosols! He was wrong about masks and lockdowns, the IFR, etc. Talk about misinformation... and from that platform...

To add "insult to injury", if you will, Dr. Gupta took part in promoting the vaccines to small children. This was nine months after we knew they didn't prevent anyone from getting or spreading the disease. They used Big Bird to help children overcome their fear of needles. Never mind that this was an experimental injection about which no one knew the long term side effects. We did, however, know about myocarditis in older children.

This was one of the lowest points in the entire pandemic. Athletes were keeling over on the soccer pitch and Dr. Gupta was pushing these injections into small children using Sesame Street characters to make them feel comfortable. Erica Hill, too. Sick, evil, call it what you want. Children this age have a one-in-a-million chance of dying with or from this infection. The vaccines don't even work. Look at the data from the trials. Giving these vaccines to children in this age group does not benefit them. It only exposes them to unknown side effects. How could Sanjay Gupta and Erica Hill have agreed to abuse children in this way?

11. **Daniel Andrews** Premier of Victoria, Australia Directed Ruthless punishment toward anyone who violated the draconian measures he put in place During COVID-19 Among the most cruel in the world

‘Sesame Street’ characters are getting their COVID-19 vaccines

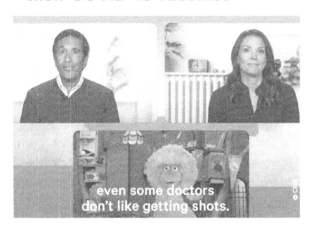

even some doctors don't like getting shots.

11. Peter Hotez, M.D., PhD

12. Jonathan Reiner, M.D.

13. Ashish Jha, M.D. MPH

14. Joe Biden

Saying "if you get the vaccine, you can't get infected" caused hundreds of thousands to get infected and hundreds to die, possibly thousands. Forcing the armed services and businesses with over 100 employees to require vaccination of their ranks will cause hundreds to die.

15. WHO Director Tedros

16. William Haseltine, PhD

17. Karl Lauterbach, Federal Minister of Health, Germany

The most bizarre statements have come out of Dr. Lauterbach's mouth.

all the way up to September 11, 2021, he said, "This is a pandemic of the unvaccinated." Even President Biden and Drs. Walensky and Fauci weren't saying it *that* late! Or were they…?

18. Anderson Cooper

Numbers 18 – 23. Wrong about almost everything.

19. Don Lemon

20. Chris Cuomo

21. Chris Hayes

22. Jake Tapper

Jake! Your parents are reported to be a doctor and nurse. How could you be so wrong on everything. Consult them next time!

23. John King

Those weren't new confirmed cases, John. They were positive PCR tests which meant almost nothing. He was ginning up fear in the population, causing the public to accept lockdowns, etc which killed or will kill 150 million innocent souls at least..

27 Who Signed Peter Daszak's Lancet Letter Denouncing as a Conspiracy Theory, the Possibility that the Virus Came From a Lab

The point of this list is to show how easily grown up professional people can be hoodwinked into taking part in a cover-up of something as important as the origin of a virus that was spreading throughout the word and killing masses of people. The letter:

Statement in support of the scientists, public health professionals, and medical professionals of China combating COVID-19

February 19, 2020 (on February 20, 2020 not knowing about this letter, I made a post in Facebook, proving that the virus came from a lab.)

We are public health scientists who have closely followed the emergence of 2019 novel coronavirus disease (COVID-19) and are deeply concerned about its impact on global health and wellbeing. We have watched as the scientists, public health professionals, and medical professionals of China, in particular, have worked diligently and effectively to rapidly identify the pathogen behind this outbreak, put in place significant measures to reduce its impact, and share their results transparently with the global health community. This effort has been remarkable.

We sign this statement in solidarity with all scientists and health professionals in China who continue to save lives and protect global health during the challenge of the COVID-19 outbreak. We are all in this together, with our Chinese counterparts in the forefront, against this new viral threat.

The rapid, open, and transparent sharing of data on this outbreak is now being threatened by rumors and misinformation around its origins. We stand together to strongly condemn conspiracy theories suggesting that COVID-19 does not have a natural origin. Scientists from multiple countries have published and analyzed genomes of the causative agent, severe acute respiratory syndrome coronavirus 2 (SARS-CoV-2),[1] and they overwhelmingly conclude that this coronavirus originated in wildlife,[2, 3, 4, 5, 6, 7, 8, 9, 10] as have so many other emerging pathogens.[11, 12] This is further supported by a letter from the presidents of the US National Academies of Science, Engineering, and Medicine[13] and by the scientific communities they represent. Conspiracy theories do nothing but create fear, rumors, and prejudice that jeopardize our global collaboration in the fight against this virus. We support the call from the Director-General of WHO to promote scientific evidence and unity over misinformation and conjecture. We want you, the science and health professionals of China, to know that we stand with you in your fight against this virus.

We invite others to join us in supporting the scientists, public health professionals, and medical professionals of Wuhan and across China. Stand with our colleagues on the frontline!

The signers:

1. Charles Calisher, 2. Dennis Carroll, 3. Rita Colwell, 4. Ronald B Corley, 5. Peter Daszak, 6. Christian Drosten, 7. Luis Enjuanes, 8. Jeremy Farrar, 9. Hume Field, 10. Josie Golding, 11. Alexander Gorbalenya 12. Bart Haagmans, 13. James M Hughes, 14. William B Karesh, 15. Gerald T Keusch, 16. Sai Kit Lam, 17. Juan Lubroth, 18. John S Mackenzie, 19. Larry Madoff, 20. Jonna Mazet, 21. Peter Palese, 22. Stanley Perlman, 23. Leo Poon, 24. Bernard Roizman, 25. Linda Saif, 26. Kanta Subbarao, 27. Mike Turner

This is one of the most shocking documents of the pandemic. Look at a few statements from this letter, published in one of the two or three most prestigious medical journals in the world, signed by people who claim to be leading public health scientists.

1. "The rapid, open, and transparent sharing of data on this outbreak is now being threatened by rumors and misinformation around its origins. We stand together to strongly condemn conspiracy theories suggesting that COVID-19 does not have a natural origin."

2. "Scientists from multiple countries have published and analyzed genomes of the causative agent, severe acute respiratory syndrome coronavirus 2 (SARS-CoV-2), and they overwhelmingly conclude that this coronavirus originated in wildlife."

Those scientists from multiple countries must be incredibly incompetent. I've looked at the genome too and the phrase "man-made" screams aloud. No reasonable person, let alone someone who calls him or herself a scientist, could come to any other conclusion and I said so in a post on February 20, 2020. In fact, I proved it to a degree of epistemic certainty equal to 10^{114} to 1 based on the lack of an intermediate stage in the steps required for a pandemic to occur and on the same order based on inserts in the genome that could not be present due to mutation or recombination. My analysis is no conspiracy theory. It is a mathematical analysis of the chances this genome could have arisen from natural zoonotic spillover and the answer is a one grain of sand from all the beaches in the world equals a big fat zero. Arithmetic was all I used, suggesting that these people need to go back to the third grade. Most people have heard about the furin cleavage site and that is compelling evidence of man's involvement but it is only the tip of the iceberg. There is a veritable treasure trove of out of left field sequences in that genome.

It comes back to the same question. Are these people, evil, corrupt, incompetent, cowards, blinded by political ideology or what? I've thought this through the many times I do one of these analyses of something that is so absurd, it is beyond the threshold of stupidity- YouTube not allowing a video to say "Hydroxychloroquine is safe", or Anthony Fauci, Atul Guwande and others claiming that the immunity conferred by those horrible vaccines is superior to that which one gains from getting and recovering from the disease, or Bill Gates suggesting in October of 2020 that we need more contact tracing for a respiratory virus that can stay in the air for days or here, where the lab origin position is called a conspiracy theory by public health scientists and geneticists who have looked at a genome that has man's fingerprints all over it.

I keep coming to the conclusion that it is a combination of all of those things. There are evil people who have been involved since the beginning. I already showed there was planning beforehand. They recruit incompetent and corrupt scientists to write journal articles that support the Narrative. There are cowards who see this happening but do not speak up as people, even small children, are dying because of it. And there are people whose political ideology has taken over their ability to think straight and twisted it into a kind of "end justifies the means" philosophy that placates their consciences as in, "well, I know the virus was created by someone in a lab, and that the vaccines and lockdowns have sent the all-cause mortality through the roof, but to admit these things would go against the superior outcome of government control over people for the good of mankind in the long run."

Sure, it makes no sense to me and many of you who are reading this book, but it makes perfect sense to a lot of people out there trying to change the political systems of the West into communist utopias. Yes, the term "communist utopia" is an oxymoron, but just look at how successful the people who are striving for this have been recently in Canada, New Zealand, even Australia and some parts of Europe? It's the "you'll own nothing and be happy" crowd and they are not to be written off as the "J.V team". This is a life and death struggle for existence the way we know it.

How could so many public health scientists be so unscientific about an issue of such great importance to public health? I'm not familiar with any of these names except, of course, #5 Peter Daszak and #8 Jeremy Farrar, both of whom were heavily involved in the cover-up of the virus's origin from a lab.

At the close of this Lancet letter was the statement, "We declare no competing interests". Yeah, right. This letter, in fact, was. arranged by Peter Daszak and Jeremy Farrar helped Anthony Fauci arrange the conference call among several scientists involved in the cover-up of the origin of the virus, the evening before the "Proximal Origins" paper was written by Kristian Andersen, Robert Garry, Andrew Rambaut, Ian Lipkin, and Edward Holmes. "Our analyses clearly show that SARS-CoV-2 is not a laboratory construct or a purposefully manipulated virus", they wrote in the paper (published in Nature) even though the day before, Andersen told Dr. Fauci in an email, "after discussions earlier today, Eddie, Bob, Mike, and myself all find the genome inconsistent with expectations from evolutionary theory." What happened in between? After the paper was published, two of the participants received huge increases in their funding

10 Politicians Most Brave in Challenging "The Narrative"

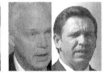

1. **Stefan Lofven, Prime Minister of Sweden**
2. **Rand Paul, M.D., U.S. Senator R-KY**
3. **Ron Johnson, U.S.Senator R-WI**
2. **Ron DeSantis, Florida Governor**
4. **Greg Abbot, Texas Governor**

With Reeves, below, correctly stopped mask mandates and opened for business when the M.D.T.V. Mafia saying it was going to be a disaster, Joe Biden saying it was "Neanderthal Thinking" and Gavin Newsome saying it was "reckless behavior". Abbot and Reeves were right. The cases continued to drop.

5. **Tate Reeves, Mississippi Governor**
6. **Tom Cotton, U.S. Senator**
7. **Christine Anderson, European Parliament**

"Bravery is actually what it takes. Courage is what it takes to stand in the way of the globalist elites because they are unscrupulous and they will do whatever they can. This vaccine campaign will go down as the biggest scandal in medical history and, moreover, it will be known as the biggest crime ever committed on humanity."

10. **Mislav Kolacusic, European Parliament**

I never thought I'd be siding with a guy named Mislav over the Prime Minister of Canada when it comes to the question of communism, but that is exactly what I'm doing.

17 Best Data Interpreters

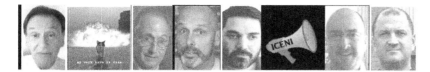

This one of the most prestigious categories and one of the most competitive

T1. Norman Fenton, PhD

T1. El Gato Malo

T1. Michael Levitt, PhD

T1. Ivor Cummins

T5. Alexandros Marinos

T5. Spartacus

T5. Harold (of World)

T6. Ah Khan Syed, M.D., PhD

T6. Toby Rogers, PhD

T7. Prashant Pradhan

T7. Jikkyleaks

T7. Igor Chudov

17. Mathew Crawford

14. John Ioannidis, M.D.

Dr. Ioannidis would rate higher if it wasn't for two errors in thinking I believe he is guilty of. In an interview with Vinay Prasad, M.D., MPH, Dr. Ioannidis stated that he believed surgical masks were 10% effective in reducing SARS-2 transmission. From the conversation, I gathered that he based this on the results from the Bangladesh Study which was fraught with difficulties.

There is so much evidence indicating that surgical masks do not reduce the spread of respiratory viruses significantly that I believe this is a very rare case where Dr. Ioannidis is wrong. I wonder whether he recognized that there was clear bias in selecting a key treated group or whether he interpreted the data incorrectly.

The other instance where I think Dr. Ioannidis probably misinterpreted the data was when he concluded from a meta-analysis he performed, that HCQ shows no benefit as a prophylactic or treating agent. Again, I think there is far too much evidence that it shows non-zero efficacy as both a prophylactic and treating agent.

I'm sure Dr. Ioannidis would never do this but I've noticed that many HCQ and Ivermectin skeptics have based their position on the conclusions of the numerous papers that have been written instead of looking at the data generated.

15. Tracey Hoeg, M.D., PhD

16. Vinay Prasad, M.D., MPH

17. Jessica Rose, PhD

17 Laymen Who Entered the Fray Very Much to Their Utter Humiliation

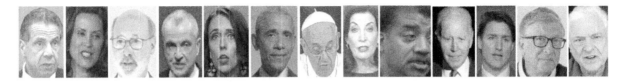

1. Andrew Cuomo, New York Governor

His administration forced nursing homes to readmit people sick with COVID-19, back from hospitals where they were being treated. Over 9,000 such patients were sent back to the stagnant air of hundreds of such nursing homes where vulnerable fellow residents waited. (please see #s 2, 3, and 4). This spread disease and caused deaths. The Cuomo administration tried to cover up the impact of this colossal failure of policy by underreporting nursing home deaths by about one-half. We'll never know the exact number of deaths this caused. The sad thing is that it was entirely unnecessary. They did it to make room for less vulnerable admits into what turned out to be relatively empty hospitals. The white mercy ships called in to provide beds in the coming overflow sat in New York Harbor for a few weeks and left when it was clear they were not needed.

2. Gretchen Whitmer, Michigan Governor

(See no. 1)

3. Tom Wolf, Pennsylvania Governor

(See no. 1)

4. Phil Murphy, New Jersey Governor

(See no. 1)

5. Jacinda Ardern, New Zealand Prime Minister

Gloating about success is never a good idea when you don't know why it happened. NZ is getting crushed now. Their early success was not due to anything Jacinda Ardern put in place. It was due to NZ being an island nation in the southern hemisphere. It was summertime when the initial wave hit. With only one main international airport due to its tiny size, it was easy to block incoming carriers. All of this only delayed the inevitable, of course. Ardern's failures have been at tremendous cost to the citizens of New Zealand. Draconian measures rivaling those of neighboring Australia- strict lockdowns, and mask enforcement, in particular- caused profound pain and mistrust of leadership that they will be feeling the effects of for a very long time.

Ardern was also caught on video telling a guest of hers on the podium to put on a mask for show

6. Barack Obama

Images of former President Obama sitting in grammar school classrooms urging children to get the vaccine will be forever etched in the memories of Americans. It's understandable that Obama would make a mistake like this, not knowing anything about medicine, and that's precisely why he should have refused to weigh in on health matters. It never ends well when politicians play doctor. Ask Andrew Cuomo.

7. Pope Francis

8. Kathy Hochul N.Y. Governor (replaced Andrew Cuomo)

9. Neil De Grasse Tyson, PhD

Wrong about masks, vaccines and lockdowns. You would have thought he might have understood the implications of a 100 nm virus but like almost everyone else, he did not.

10. Joe Biden

I'll just bring up two instances here. He gets beat up constantly over his misunderstanding of SARS-2 science. His mental state makes it almost impossible for him to comprehend the movements of a set of viruses that have baffled those who have their faculties intact but support the Narrative. Biden has made his misunderstanding known on almost a daily basis. When Texas Governor Greg Abbott decided to lift the mask mandates in March of 2021, and let everyone go back to work, President Biden announced that "It was Neanderthal thinking." He was wrong, of course. It was exactly what needed to be done. Mask mandates and business closures should never have been enacted in the first place.

In March, 2021, Abbott stopped the mask mandates and let businesses open. The cases continued to drop at the same rate because masks and mandates had nothing to do with why the cases were dropping in the first place. The descent was due to the fact that we had reached herd immunity on January 11, 2021. That's why, when March came and went, nothing changed. Mask mandates, lockdowns (including business closures and school closures) never reduced the ascending slope of cases, hospitalizations, or deaths vs. time for any country at any time. The myth of "flattening the curve" was just that; a myth.

The second example consists of Biden's insistence that if you've been vaccinated, you are protected from getting the virus. Biden repeatedly misled the public regarding the inability of the vaccines to block transmission of the virus. He said over and over that "if you are vaccinated, you can't pass this on to another person". He said this at least into August of 2021 when I had proved in mid-January that the vaccine was not preventing spread. In fairness to Biden, Drs. Fauci and Walensky were saying the same thing into June at least. I don't think many people would have taken the vaccine if they knew it wasn't blocking transmission. Fauci and Walensky probably couldn't have figured this out in January, but by April they should have known and stopped misleading the public on such a life and death issue. We don't know why they continued to mislead the public.

11. Justin Trudeau Prime Minister of Canada

Aside from all the things he has done so far during his tenure as PM of Canada that has them moving inexorably toward a socialist/communist state, his attempts at playing doctor displayed a most profound misunderstanding of medical science. This has been matched by only Andrew Cuomo before he stepped down as Governor of New York. Here's a quote of Trudeau's, delivered on August 27, 2021: "Vaccines are the best way to finish the fight against COVID-19. That's why we will make vaccines mandatory for anyone boarding a plane or train, or any federally-regulated worker. This is how we will keep everyone, including our kids, safe and healthy."

This statement makes sense only if the vaccine was able to prevent the spread of the virus. It wasn't and Trudeau should have known it. I had proved this seven months earlier. Everyone knew this by late August except, evidently, for Trudeau, Karl Lauterbach of Germany, and Joe Biden

Trudeau was putting children at greater risk by mandating all other passengers be vaccinated if, for no other reason than the vaccinated incorrectly thinking they could breathe into another person's face for a long flight without consequences, a sense of false security if you will. I addressed this very question in a video I made on January 24, 2021 about a week after I had proved that the vaccines were not blocking transmission. I used data out of Israel since they were getting doses into arms faster than we were in the U.S. It was "absurdly illogical ", I said, to require people to be vaccinated before they got on a plane with a vaccine that didn't block transmission. The degree of stupidity associated with this thing was and still is mind boggling. When considering the harm these policies placed on the ordinary citizen and on society in general, you have to think they were done with the full knowledge that they would not do anything positive while causing the virus to spread faster. The policies they chose were simply below the threshold where one could enact them out of stupidity.

12. Bill Gates

In October of 2020, Bill said we were not doing as well as other countries on contact tracing and needed to step up our efforts. This was not the most intelligent thing he has ever said. Once a respiratory virus transmitted by aerosols is out in a population, contact tracing is futile. There were doctors, such as Jonathan Reiner, who believed as Gates did but they were wrong too. Contract tracing works well for something like AIDS because you can remember who you have been intimate with, but there's no way you'd know who exhaled the virus that you inhaled in an office building or a grocery store. Aerosols can stay in the air for hours or even days.

13. Art Caplan, PhD

Dr. Caplan has a PhD in the History and Philosophy of Science and works on problems of medical ethics. He is the Head of the Division of Biomedical Ethics at the NYU School of Medicine. I'm shocked every time I hear him speak. His knowledge of the medical science behind COVID-19 is quite limited. On top of this, he says things like: "It's OK for doctors to refuse to treat the unvaccinated". Is he saying unvaccinated patients should be punished? Is he trying to protect the practitioner? The first is unethical. The second displays a profound misunderstanding of the transmission profile for the virus and its variants. I believe the first explanation is the reason he thinks it's OK for doctors to refuse to treat the unvaccinated. Just about every position I've heard him take is unethical. Well into 2022, he still believes masks work, and encourages people to get the vaccines and boosters.

14. Randi Weingarten

President of the American Federation of Teachers, she pushed Rochelle Walensky and the CDC to keep schools closed. The teachers, who were getting paid while they were not working, were very happy. Students paid an enormous price for this theft of taxpayer money. They will drop out of school at a higher rate, be more likely to live in poverty, earn less than if they had not had their education interrupted, and live shorter lives. Parents are finding out about the influence Weingarten had in directing policy at the CDC and are furious. It wasn't about science. It was about politics and money.

15. Bill Nye

He's popular from a children's show called "Bill Nye, the Science Guy". In his earlier life, he was a mechanical engineer and a stand-up comedian. He performed an experiment of sorts I saw on the internet, trying to blow out a candle with various types of masks and concluded that masks are helpful. The problem is, surgical masks, for example, direct lots of the exhaust out the sides. It still infects people around you even though the candle doesn't get blown out as easily as if you didn't have a mask on. He could have saved himself this embarrassment if he had just checked the literature. And you can't mandate N95 masks. People can't even tolerate surgical masks. N95 masks need to be fitted and have a tight seal around the periphery to produce a minimal benefit if any. People can't stand them. In minutes, the seal gets broken. N95 mandates? Forget it

16. Beto O'Rourke

Another bizarre statement from someone who should know the damage their words cause. In March, 2021, again, O'Rourke announced that "Abbott is killing the people of Texas" and the decision to stop the mask mandates and open up Texas for business was "a death warrant for Texans." He was wrong, of course. The problem with O'Rourke and Biden is that they don't understand how the characteristics of a virus that is 100 nanometers in diameter relate to whether wearing a surgical or cloth mask will reduce its spread. O'Rourke doesn't know anything about science. Evidently his advisors, if he has any, didn't either. If he did have someone helping him on this, he should have asked him or her, "Is there any chance the cases aren't going to rebound when Abbott lifts the restrictions because if the cases keep going down I'm going to look like an idiot?" O'Rourke either didn't have that conversation or he needs a new advisor.

It's worth pointing out that O'Rourke was not alone. Everybody jumped on the bandwagon including some medical doctors who should have known better. However, by this point, it was clear that they were wrong on almost everything. Dr Fauci said, "It is ill-advised for Abbott to lift the mask mandates". Dr. Reiner said, "We've seen this movie and it doesn't turn out well." Gavin Newsome said it was "absolutely reckless to remove the mask mandates". Joe Biden said removing the mask mandates and opening up Texas was "Neanderthal thinking". As expected for anyone who understands that masks don't do a thing and that opening up for business probably reduces the number of people getting COVID because it gets people out of the stagnant air in their houses, cases in Texas didn't just stay the same, they decreased.

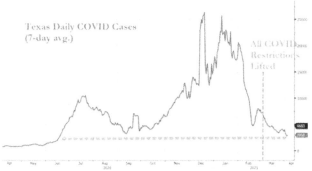

Trevor Noah weighed in as a comedian when he said "We shouldn't do whatever the 'F' Texas is doing." Comedians get a pass and should. But Noah clearly showed himself to be wrong in serious conversations and is ranked in the category of late night and other comedians who were aggressive in pushing the fear narrative. These people can always say "What do I know? I'm a comedian." The problem is, they have big platforms and their followers think that because they are on television, they know things. Those followers believe that if someone is famous, they know more than the average Joe English major, which O'Rourke is. This is a common misunderstanding. It's why the voices of actors are given too much weight when they endorse something like CO_2 being the primary driver of climate change. Leo DiCaprio is an outstanding actor, truly exceptional, but he doesn't understand the forces at play in determining whether fossil fuel use is the major contributor to or even a significant driver of climate change. He definitely should not be speaking to the UN Assembly on this topic. I shouldn't be too hard on DiCaprio. He's voicing his opinion and we need more, not less of that. But the public should put absolutely no weight behind it when they find out that he doesn't have the slightest idea what he is talking about, and why should he?

The amazing thing about the SARS-2 debacle is not that the Leo DiCaprios of the world who don't have any background in the subject and consequently do not understand the science behind COVID-19, it's that many scientists who have made this subject matter their life's work and are involved with it every day, don't understand this either. I'm talking about epidemiologists, researchers in the fields of virology, vaccine-ology, immunology, etc.- some of whom lecture about this in Universities and appear on television as experts, or who work as everyday clinical doctors. The great majority of these people have done much worse than flipping a coin. In other words, you would have been better off believing the exact opposite of everything they said.

People, including doctors, shouldn't speak up unless they have a sound argument behind their claims and predictions and they should present the argument at the same time that they make those claims. Most importantly, they should be called out when they're wrong because peoples' lives are at stake and millions of people died because of their mistakes or the purposeful misleading of the public. This is the only way we're going to make our society better.

Just a few weeks ago, the VRBPAC (please see list of committee members elsewhere) authorized the use of the Moderna and Pfizer mRNA vaccines in babies only six months of age. This decision was not justified based on the trials that were undertaken. It's hard to believe these people are this inept. Or has corruption gotten to them? Is it possible for a person to be so depraved that he or she would put their bank accounts above the lives of innocent babies? Are there nefarious goings-on behind the scenes that we get peeks of, now and then? I happen to think there are. It's the only way I can explain the entirety of this mess.

17. Rena Conti, PhD, Boston University Associate Professor of Business (marketing)

In an interview dated January 31, 2022, she stated, "What we know is that there are no studies that suggest ivermectin is effective at treating COVID-19." No, you don't know that because there are many studies in the literature from all over the world that show ivermectin is effective at treating COVID-19. I'll help you. Here's a meta-analysis showing a 62% reduction in the risk of death (treatment) and an 86% reduction in the risk of getting the disease (prophylaxis) published in the July/August, 2021 edition of the American Journal of Therapeutics. You had plenty of time to review this meta-analysis before you wrote your paper:

https://journals.lww.com/americantherapeutics/Fulltext/2021/08000/Ivermectin_for_Prevention_and_Treatment_of.7.aspx

10 *Brave Women*

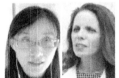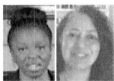

1. Li-Meng Yan, M.D., PhD
2. Simone Gold, M.D., J.D.
4. Ngozi Ezike, M.D.
5. Sunetra Gupta, PhD
6. Tess Lawrie, MBBCh, PhD
7. Mary Talley Bowden, M.D
8. Jessica Rose, PhD
9. Dr. Clare Craig
10. Stella Emanuel, M.D.

10 New COVID-19 Billionaires

The "old" Billionaires involved in social media and e-commerce profited much more than the 10 listed below. Even Bill Gates' $55 M investment in September of 2019 in BioNTech, an obscure German biotech company, not trading publicly at the time, returned 10 - 30x in two years, virtually unheard of for a biotech company. Most of the new billionaires got wealthy off of products like masks and vaccines that did not work. A large fraction of the masks are now floating in our oceans.

1. **Li Jianquan (Hong Kong),** Masks and PPE $6.8 Billion
2. **Stephane Bancel (France),** Moderna CEO $4.3 Billion
3. **Liu Fangyi (China),** Masks, Hand Sanitizer $4.2 Billion
4. **Uğur Şahin (Germany),** BioNTech CEO $4 Billion
5. **Dai Lizhong (China),** The FDA authorized Sansure Diagnostics testing kits in May of 2020 $2.4 Billion
6. **Tim Springer (USA),** Harvard Professor. 3.5% of Moderna $2.2 Billion
7. **Sergio Stevanato (Italy)** Supplied glass vials for COVID vaccines $1.9 Billion
8. **Noubar Afeyan (USA),** Co-founder of Moderna $1.9 Billion
9. **Juan Lopez (Spain),** Packaged vaccines for Moderna $1.8 Billion
10. **Robert Langer (USA),** M.I.T. Professor 3% stake, Co- founder of Moderna $1.6 Billion

8 Japanese Villains

Japanese people suffered because of cultural restrictions. Being an individual who goes against the crowd is frowned upon in Japanese society. Many who disagreed with the masking policies (and others) knew they were unfounded but "went along anyway".

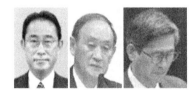

1. **Fumio Kishida**
2. **Yoshihide Suga**
3. **Shegeru Omi**
4. **Yoshihito Niki**
   Refuses to unmask the population until Japan reaches an absurd boosted threshold
5. **Kotaro Nagasaki**- called on residents not fully vaccinated to refrain from going out
6. **Shinji Harai**- mask pushing with no justification
7. **Hideaki Omura**
8. **Taro Komo**-

34 Members of the FDA'a Vaccines and Related Biological Products Advisory Committee (VRBPAC) and the CDC's Advisory Committee on Immunization Practices (ACIP)

The Study Used to Gain Approval for Children 5 – 11 was laughable. There were 1,518 in the treated group and 750 in the control group, all w/o prior evidence of SARS-2 infection. Why did they use such a tiny number of participants for a disease with a one-in-a-million chance of dying "with" or "from" covid-19? As expected, there were zero cases of severe COVID and zero cases of death in both groups. Since children recover easily from mild and moderate disease, there was no basis for asking to be granted "Emergency" Use Authorization, based on this study.

But the real harm in using these low numbers is in hiding adverse effects from the vaccines which occur at a much higher rate than death. The FDA asked Pfizer to increase their numbers early in the trial. Pfizer used data from another study (patients were a different age) but in this study, they followed the patients for only 17 days. In their own trial, they only followed patients for two months. (Many adverse outcomes from vaccines, such as cancer and auto-immune disorders, take much longer to develop. Pfizer eliminated these possibilities by making their follow-up periods very short.)

Why did they use patients with no evidence of prior infection? To eliminate the chance that the vaccine would damage their natural immunity (according to data from Great Britain that showed the vaccine interferes with your ability to form antibodies against the "non-spike" proteins of the virus, such as the nucleocapsid proteins in the viral capsule, reducing the long-term protection afforded by natural immunity and making recipients more vulnerable to mutations in the mRNA coding for the spike proteins. In order to eliminate the risk for Pfizer of something like this happening, just limit the study to those who have not been infected by SARS-2.

The risk-benefit model used by the FDA only considered one adverse outcome- myocarditis- which tends to occur in older patients. No other adverse outcomes were considered, even short-term conditions like anaphylaxis. And obviously, long-term conditions weren't considered. Since no one in either group experienced any adverse effects (due to the low numbers in the trial and the extremely short follow-up), how can they claim "90% effectiveness" (Walensky) for the vaccines in reducing the chance of infection? They arrived at this number by looking at the antibody titers in the blood of trial participants in another study involving 16 to 25-year-olds, and measured what level of antibodies prevented cases, hospitalizations and deaths. Then they assumed there was an analogous level in 5 – 11-year-olds that was protective and used that to arrive at the figure of "90% effective" in preventing these things. The chutzpah of these Big Pharma executives in thinking they could get this junk science by anyone but the corrupt, is astounding.

The risk benefit profile generated from this study is deeply flawed because it does not take into account that cardiac damage is cumulative and everyone agrees that the vaccines only last 4 – 6 months. To publicize the adverse event risk over only 6 months is flat out wrong. These children will have to take a shot twice a year.

Looking at the numbers… There are 28,384,878 children aged 5 – 11 in the US. Using the FDA's estimate that there will be 106 excess myocarditis cases (due to the vaccine) per million, we will see 3009 new cases every six months. But what about those kids who came in just under the myocarditis threshold in their last six months? Since the damage is cumulative, they will get myocarditis too and would have to be added to the 3009. And the third 6-month period, and the fourth 6-month period, and the... PLUS the myocarditis itself is progressively deadly. Whatever the number dead out of ten after two years, it is greater after four.

These are the people who approved the vaccines in children without any justification. If you see them in the grocery store, ask them how they could have justified EUA approval when no one in either group got seriously ill.

VRBPAC:
1. **Hana El Sahly, M.D. , Chair**
2. **Hayley Altman-Gans, M.D.**
3. **Paula Annunziato, M.D. *****
4. **Adam C. Berger, Ph.D.**
5. **Henry H. Bernstein, D.O., MHCM, FAAP**
6. **Archana Chatterjee, M.D., Ph.D.**
7. **CAPT Amanda Cohn, M.D.**
8. **Holly Janes, Ph.D.**
9. **David Kim, M.D., M.S., M.H.A.**
10. **Arnold Monto, M.D.**
11. **Paul Offit, M.D.**
12. **Steven Pergam, M.D.**
13. **Jay Portnoy, M.D.**
14. **Eric J. Rubin, M.D., Ph.D.**
15. **Andrea Shane, M.D., M.P.H., M.Sc.**
16. **Gregg Sylvester, M.D., M.P.H. +**
17. **Sussan Paydar, Ph.D.**
18. **Lashawn Marks, COMMITTEE MANAGEMENT SPECIALIST**
19. **Prabhakara Atreya, Ph.D., DIRECTOR**

ACIP:

1. **Kevin A. Ault, MD, FACOG, FIDSA**
2. **Lynn Bahta, RN, MPH, CPH**
3. **Beth P. Bell, MD, MPH**
4. **Oliver Brooks, MD, FAAP**
5. **Wilbur H. Chen, MD, MS, FIDSA, FACP**
6. **Sybil Cineas, MD, FAAP, FACP**
7. **Matthew F. Daley, MD**
8. **Camille N. Kotton, MD, FIDSA, FAST**
9. **James Loehr, MD, FAAFP**
10. **Grace M. Lee, MD, MPH**
11. **Sarah S. Long, MD**
12. **Veronica V. McNally, J.D.**
13. **Katherine A. Poehling, MD, MPH**

14. **Pablo J. Sanchez, M.D.**
15. **Helen Keipp Talbot, MD, MPH**

13 People Who Think in Principles

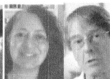

People who think in principles are frequently the ones who make accurate predictions. People who think in principles don't change their minds often because the principles they used in coming up with their original positions do not change. If data comes in that clearly disproves their original theory, they go back to examine their reasoning and find the error(s). They will humbly disclose where they went wrong. Again, this is rare because they base their positions on reasoning.

As an example, a person thinking in principles would consider the question of whether mask use in the community would significantly reduce the spread of a respiratory virus like SARS-2 in the following way: He/She would recognize that the relative sizes of the particle and the openings in the material being penetrated is a fundamental. He would know his basic facts about these sizes. He would know that there are enormous gaps on the sides of surgical masks. He might do a quick thought experiment where the subject inhales smoke from a cigarette and exhales by talking or blowing and see in his mind that the particulates come through the mask and around it. This, coupled with the knowledge that the particulates in smoke are much larger than the virus particles (which are so small, they're invisible) tells him that masks cannot block virus particles expelled on one's breath as aerosols. He would consider special cases and determine whether they are significant; cases such as the spread that results from the particles expelled when a person sneezes or "wet coughs". He knows that in such cases, masks would definitely trap most of the water droplets covered with virus. That's something in favor of mask use. Is it significant?

Quickly realizing that almost all people turn away from others around them and cover their mouths and noses when they sneeze or cough, and doing a quick comparison of the number of times one breathes in a day vs. the number of times they sneeze or cough, he comes to the conclusion that sneezing and coughing are a negligible way in which this virus gets transmitted from person to person. Just to make sure, he tries to think of the last time someone sneezed or wet-coughed in his face. Realizing that he could be forgetting some, he can't remember a single time. Then he realizes an amusing byproduct of sneezing with a surgical mask on- that when one sneezes after he has turned his face reflexively 90 degrees to the left or right and put his hands in front of the mask, the water droplets fly out the sides of the mask, directly into the person's face he was turning away from. He might also think of an analogous situation with other diseases that could be transmitted by wet-coughing or sneezing.

Gonorrhea is caused by a bacterium, Neisseria gonorrhea, that resides in the throat and oropharynx in addition to other, more obvious places in the body. It's definitely possible that one could transmit gonorrhea by wet coughing or sneezing into another person's face (nose and mouth). Do we all walk around in masks to prevent ourselves from catching gonorrhea? No, we don't. We don't because, while this is certainly possible, it is a negligible way in which this bacterium is transmitted. And it's the

80

same with COVID-19. Transmission of the SARS-2 virus by wet coughing or sneezing is a negligible way in which it is transmitted. Mask wearing by those in the community is simply a solution for a problem that does not exist, namely the significant transmission of SARS-2 by wet-coughing or sneezing (and, of course, we know, and our "thinker in principles" would know, the cough that accompanies SARS-2 infection is dry, not wet.). He figured out all of this without seeing a single piece of data, just by reasoning from first principles. But then, out of curiosity, he searches the literature and finds an NIH paper that confirms his reasoning. Looking at 72 years of meta-analyses covering randomized-controlled trials, in not a single instance, did the use of surgical face masks significantly reduce transmission of laboratory-confirmed influenza. I would add that because those who reason from first principles do not generally need data to figure out what is happening, they are invariably the ones who predict correctly the behavior of a virus or the course of a pandemic before a single database is created or graph is drawn. I am very lucky that this way of thinking is part of my nature and then it was honed as a physics major at M.I.T. where this kind of thinking is crucial to survival. It is without question the reason why I was the first or only person to make insights and predictions on more than 22 issues of major importance regarding the SARS-2 virus, COVID-19 and the vaccines when there is not a single other person who did so on more than two issues. And as far as I can gather, I am the only person who has been right on everything so far.

People who think in principles are very rare in the field of medicine and thus our list is short. Here is an incomplete list in no particular order, of people who think in principles.

1. **El Gato Malo**
1. **Sunetra Gupta, PhD**
1. **Mike Yeadon, PhD**
1. **Martin Kulldorff, PhD**
1. **Richard Ebright, PhD**
1. **Spartacus**
1. **Matthew B. Crawford**
1. **Steve Kirsch**
1. **Peter Doshi, PhD**
1. **Jeffrey Tucker**
1. **Bill Gates**
   I think there's plenty of evidence Bill thinks this way generally, but he's done things that speak
   against it, such as thinking that contact tracing would help, eight months into a respiratory
   pandemic. Or that COVID-19 at any time indicated that it was "the once in a century pandemic we've
been waiting for".
1.**Freddie Sayers**
1.**Alex Berenson**

33 Individuals Whose Reputations Took the Biggest Hit

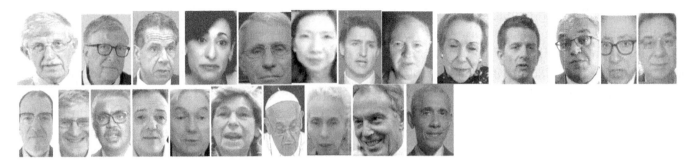

1. Francis Collins, M.D., PhD

Dr. Collins headed the U.S. arm of the Human Genome Project. He was a giant in the field of molecular biology. Then came COVID-19. As NIH Director, he approved grants to Eco Health Alliance who subcontracted gain of function research to the Wuhan Institute of Virology. Then he engaged in a cover-up, characterizing the lab leak hypothesis a "conspiracy theory". He then requested a "published takedown" of the GBD co-authors, referring to them as "fringe epidemiologists". Finally, the kickback scandal surfaced and the NIH refused to provide documents re: who received payments from whom, that is until a judge ordered them to do so. He wrecked his stellar reputation and exchanged his place in history from being one of the leaders in a worldwide effort to achieve what could be considered the greatest milestone of the 20th century in the biological sciences, to someone who did everything he could to stifle scientific debate.

2. Bill Gates

3. Andrew Cuomo

Remember when Cuomo was seriously considered as a replacement for Joe Biden on the 2024 Presidential ticket? I don't think that's going to happen anymore. It wasn't the sexual harassment claims that did him in. It was his handling of COVID-19. He started playing doctor during his nightly briefings. He actively pushed the most destructive healthcare policy ever created and explained how it would "flatten the curve" to give a break to mostly empty hospitals.

4. Rochelle Walensky, M.D.

I didn't know Dr. Walensky before she took over for Dr. Redfield as the CDC Director but she was the Chief of Infectious Disease at The Massachusetts General Hospital in Boston, one of Harvard's teaching hospitals. To be chief of anything there is prestigious. As CDC Director, she's been wrong on almost every call. Four plus months after I had established that the vaccine didn't block transmission, she was still telling the public that it did. She said she felt a sense of "impending doom " on March 29, 2021, two-and-a-half months after I showed that we had reached herd immunity for the Wuhan strain (without a single person fully-vaccinated, I might add). It seemed like she has never known what was going on and even admitted once that she didn't understand the numbers. Recently, she has pushed the vaccines in six-month-old babies based on a trial that did not offer adequate justification for it. Her reputation has taken an enormous hit.

5. Anthony Fauci, M.D.

To those in the know, his reputation took a substantial hit during his handling of the AIDS epidemic but nothing like what happened to it during COVID-19. He pushed masks which don't work, physical distancing to six feet which has no scientific basis and probably makes no sense at all for a virus transmitted by aerosols, vaccines that increase all cause mortality and don't block transmission, and told the public they needed to get the vaccine even if they had gotten COVID-19 and recovered from it. It didn't help that there are videos of him saying the exact opposite even though there are videos online of him saying the exact opposite.

All of this is on top of his involvement in Wuhan and the cover-up. Did he tell the public the vaccine blocked transmission for five months after it was clear that it didn't because he was unaware or because he did want to mislead them so they wouldn't refuse the vaccine? Either way, it was yet another reputation-killer.

6. Leana Wen, M.D.

This lady was the President of Planned Parenthood and selected as one of TIME Magazine's 100 Most Influential People of 2019. She was also wrong on almost every call regarding COVID. I give her the benefit of the doubt by using the word "almost" but I can't think of a single case where she was correct. Masks, lockdowns, school closures, giving the horrible vaccines to people who didn't come close to being on the right side of the risk/benefit analysis, etc. She was in favor of all of them. She had a regular and massive platform on CNN and caused an enormous amount of destruction of the livelihoods and health of innocent people. There is no question that the policies she endorsed resulted in the deaths of many, many people. She even got aggressive about pushing people to agree to the vaccines. She said to Chris Cuomo on CNN, "If everything is reopened, what's the carrot going to be? How are we going to incentivize people to actually get the vaccine?" For a doctor to threaten patients with losing their livelihoods unless they agree to inject an experimental "vaccine " into their bodies when she doesn't know anything about the risk/benefit for those patients is nothing less than evil.

7. Justin Trudeau

The Canadian Prime Minister had already done a lot of damage to his reputation in previous years but the last two have done him in. He went from being a fairly ineffectual leader, occasionally appearing in blackface, to someone with proven ties to communist China, a disastrous handling of the truckers' strike and cruel travel restrictions requiring useless and dangerous vaccination before Canadians could board a plane and leave the country. All of this while repeatedly demonstrating in speeches that he is thoroughly uninformed when it comes to COVID-19.

8. Peter Daszak, PhD

Records show Dr. Daszak was involved in a lot of reckless manipulation of bat coronaviruses. When it became apparent that he was up to his neck in the lab origin cover-up, he wrote the letter that was published in the Lancet and got 26 scientists to sign it. In the letter, the hypothesis that the virus came from a lab was described as a conspiracy theory.

He ran the investigation of the matter for the WHO. "Nothing to see here, move along" and was being paid by the US Department of Homeland Security to reduce misinformation regarding the virus and the disease it causes, COVID-19. Talk about irony... and he has never been called in for testimony under oath by Congress. He's a British citizen who has so far gotten away with getting the U.S. to fund his research through an NGO called the Eco Health Alliance and then trashing us in return. (See "**27Individuals Who Signed Peter Daszak's Faked Lancet Letter")**

9. Deborah Birx, M.D.

Most people didn't know her before the pandemic started or her ranking would be much higher because her reputation is shot now. She traveled during the time she asked everyone else to stay inside a la Neil Ferguson, but the biggest mistake she made was to push the lockdowns. According to her memoir, she tricked President Trump into extending them after the initial two weeks. She's responsible for a decent fraction of the 150+ million deaths caused by the idiotic policy of locking down healthy people.

10. Kristian Andersen, PhD

A once-respected researcher at the Scripps Institute, he co-wrote a paper proclaiming the virus originated through natural zoonotic spillover only a day after he told Dr. Fauci in an email that the virus had characteristics of having been engineered by humans. Finding out later that a conference call occurred during the time he changed his mind and that he received large grants from Dr. Fauci for the following year hinted of a sort of pay-for-play agreement. He needs to present evidence as to why he changed his mind. The problem: there isn't any (other than the possibility that he did it for the grant money.)

11. Ashish Jha, M.D. MPH

His reputation among doctors has been devastated even before he started in the White House. The general public may not notice the idiocy of his claims.

12. Jonathan Reiner, M.D.

13. Albert Bourla, DVM

14. Stefan Bancel

15. Dr. Andrew Hill

Watch this video: https://rumble.com/vwfia3-a-letter-to-andrew-hill-dr-tess-lawrie-oracle-films.html

16. Paul Offit, M.D.

A statement like this, written in an article will destroy your reputation in seconds: "The only strategy that will defeat the coronavirus is vaccinating the unvaccinated, wherever they live." With a vaccine made for a virus that was gone two years ago, that doesn't block transmission? Plus, not all the unvaccinated need the vaccine.

17. WHO Director Tedros

The WHO Director General misled the world when he said "This is a novel coronavirus and no one is immune to it." This is what happens when you get a person who is not a medical doctor to run the WHO. Then he botched the investigation into the origin of the virus. Asking one of the perpetrators, Peter Daszak, to participate did not help.

18. David Kessler,

The chief science officer of COVID-19 response at the U.S. Department of Health and Human Services. A big proponent of vaccinating children all the way down to six month-olds.

19. Shi Zheng Li, PhD

20. Jeremy Farrar, M.D.

Sometimes referred to as the "Bill Gates" of Great Britain because of his work with the Wellcome Trust. He helped arrange the teleconference in which deals appear to be made to get the "Proximal Origins of SARS-CoV-2" paper written; the first major effort to divert attention from the lab origin theory.

21. Tom Frieden, M.D., MPH

The former CDC Director displayed a profound lack of understanding of why non-pharmaceutical interventions could not work.

22. Peter Marks, M.D.

23. Boris Johnson

24. Michael Olsterholm, M.D.

In an interview on Joe Rogan's podcast dated March 10, 2020, Dr. Olsterholm said, "This thing **clearly** jumped from an animal species, probably the third week in November (2019), to humans," and "There is no evidence whatsoever that this was a bio-weapon or that it was accidentally released from the Wuhan lab. There's no evidence that it's an engineered bug. It's not." Imagine how I felt having written a post on February 20, 2020 explaining why that virus had to have been modified or made from scratch in a lab. I think this doctor was the first one I saw on video talking gibberish. I'm glad I saw it because it made me scrutinize everything I heard from that point on.

I thought, "Maybe he's some clinical internal medicine guy who doesn't know anything about molecular biology. Then, when writing this book, I wanted to give him another chance. I found a video from September 10, 2021. That was sufficiently far along for him to have learned something about COVOD-19, the variants, the vaccines, etc.

This time, he started out immediately saying things that were not correct: A) that we didn't know if Delta was a more severe disease than previous variants and the original Wuhan strain. Actually, we knew this already. Delta was much weaker. B) He said we weren't able to supply safe education for children. He's wrong here too. We were able to supply safe education for children. Even by September of 2020, we had the Swedish example which showed it was perfectly safe for children to be in school. I wrote a post in the summer of 2020 in which I argued the case for not closing them down in the first place. If you believe schools should have been shut down for COVID-19 and you want to be consistent, you have to shut them down every year for the flu because more morbidity and mortality occurs with the flu in the school-aged population, ages five to seventeen. It's really that simple. People, including this doctor, overreacted to this virus. Even much later in the year than this, on December 30, 2020 a survey was done that asked people, "What percentage of people who have been infected by the coronavirus needed to be hospitalized?" Forty-one percent of Democrats and 28% of Republicans answered that half or more of those infected by COVID-19 needed to be hospitalized. The actual number is 1 –2 %.

More things Dr. Olsterholm said that made no sense: 1) He said, "there is not going to be a concept of herd immunity here." Really? We had already reached herd immunity for Delta- on September 4, 2021 AND for the wild type, back in January. How could he not know this?) He said the corona variants will burn fast and burn hot and then it tends to drop off with many susceptible people still left in the area… and then another surge will come later. No. This is wrong. We haven't seen this with any variant yet. All have reached their herd immunity thresholds and dropped down. None have come back. He also keeps talking about the lack of vaccination causing increased transmission such as when he said spreading in nursing homes was due to the staff not getting vaccinated in high enough percentages. He said all of this in only the first 4 ½ minutes of a one-hour video. I stopped watching.

25. Randi Weingarten

26. Pope Francis

27. Donald Trump

Trump was taken advantage of by his COVID-19 advisors, Fauci and Birx in particular. It wasn't like him to let them do it. He also got hurt profoundly by all the bailouts he approved early in the summer of 2020 and for urging people to get the vaccine for too long after everyone knew it was a horrible product.

28. Michael Callahan

29. Robert Redfield, M.D

30. Mike Pence

Trump's COVID czar

31. Eric Feigl-Ding, DSc. (Epidemiology)

I didn't know Dr. Feigl-Ding was commenting on the pandemic until 2022. He offered his opinion frequently on Twitter from the beginning. Many things he said were not correct. He also endorses taking the vaccines even after it has been shown they are not effective at blocking transmission or reducing mortality.

32. Barbara Ferrer

Director of the L.A. County Department of Health, she is responsible for some of the most severe restrictions in the US, which resulted in countless businesses, public schools, public parks, and beaches, being shut down for several months. Ferrer also mandated the use of masks in Los Angeles County. Shutting down public parks and beaches shows she doesn't understand why lockdowns are detrimental and why you're better being outside in an open space. It's just incredible that the Director of a large county department of health wouldn't know something this simple.

33. Tony Blair

Pushed vaccines, stupidly. "It's your civic duty to get vaccinated." "We need to accelerate the vaccination of children". "For pregnant women, vaccination is safer than the disease". How many people did he kill by pushing these horrible injections. He is utterly unable to interpret data or he is as evil as they come.

34. Barack Obama

As more and more evidence comes out revealing collusion and malfeasance by the vaccine makers, Obama's endorsement of the vaccine for children and his push for black people to get the vaccine looks worse and worse. Siding with the criminal corporations is not a good look. He should have gotten some advice from someone who could see this coming. It's too late now. I do feel for Obama. He got some bad advice.

His 60th birthday party where everyone was walking around without masks after he had urged the general public to wear them didn't go over well either. The most hated politicians are those revealed to be hypocrites "For thee, not for me", and so forth. It doesn't matter that masks don't work. It's that he told everyone else to wear them and didn't do it himself or have his guests do it when cases were rising in the U.S. At first he said it was only going to be "family and close friends" when people started asking why a gathering like this was allowed when cases were on the rise. About four hundred people attended, including staff. Much to Obama's chagrin, the dozens of pictures that leaked didn't show anyone wearing a mask.

One thing that makes the hit to his reputation minimal is the fact that those who hold him in high esteem believe the non-pharmaceutical interventions worked too. Some of them actually think the problem was that we waited too *long* to go into lockdowns. I guess they'll be pushing for lockdowns hard and early next time.

6 Talk Show/Comedy Hosts Who Perpetuated the "4% IFR, Masks, Lockdowns, School Closings, Three Waves in Six Months, Natural Immunity Fades Quickly, Horse Paste" Idiocy and Must Accept Responsibility for Their Share of the Death and Destruction of Innocent People

1.   Steven Colbert
2.   Jimmie Kimmel
3.   Trevor Noah
4.   John Oliver
5.   Seth Myers
6.   Jimmy Fallon

7 Clinicians Achieving Spectacular Results Treating COVID-19

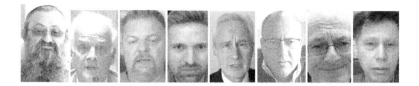

1. Vladimir "Zev" Zelenko, M.D.
2. George Fareed, M.D.

It was very magnanimous of Dr. Fareed to mention in Senate testimony that his very successful protocol was a modified version of Dr. Zelenko's protocol.

2. Brian Tyson, M.D.
4. Flavio Cadegiani, M.D. (Brasil)

 a brilliant doctor who, in high school, won gold medals in Mathematics, Physics, and Chemistry, concurrently at the Brasil Olympiad and earned his PhD in 7 months from the Universidade Federal de Sao Paolo, currently the 4th ranked university in Latin America. In roughly 4,000 patients, he had 4 hospitalizations, one intubation and no deaths.

T5. Peter McCullough, M.D., MPH
T5. Pierre Kory, M.D.
T5. Paul Marik, M.D.
T5. Harvey Risch, M.D., PhD

16 Canadian Villains

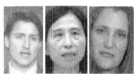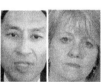

1. Justin Trudeau
2. Theresa Tam
3. Chrysta Freeland
   The deputy Prime Minister and Finance Minister of Canada is Trudeau's right hand as Canada moves toward communism hard and fast
4. Jean-Ives Duclos current Minister of Health
   There is a movement headed by PM Trudeau to redefine what it means to be fully-vaccinated in Canada.
5. Patty Hadju Minister of Health until October of 2021
   Thinks washing hands and wearing face masks reduce the spread of the virus
6. Dr. Howard Njoo
7. Dr. Margaret Gale Rowe
6. Premier Doug Ford O
7. Premier John Horgan BC
8. Dr. Bonnie Henry BC
9. Adrian Dix BC
10. Premier Jason Kennedy A
11. Dr. Deena Hinshaw A

12. **Premier Scott Moe S**
13. **Dr. Saqib Sahab S**
14. **Premier Brian Pallister M**
15. **Dr. Brent Roussin public health officer M**
16. **Tara Moriarty, PhD**

This ID/Researcher on the faculty Dentistry at the U. of Toronto believes that the spike in deaths that occurred in the second half of 2021 was due to missed Covid deaths due to inadequate testing and tracking. "The overlap is almost perfect in time. So that's a really important clue that a lot of it is likely COVID related," she said. We still don't know what caused that huge spike in deaths that has continued into 2022. Figuring out why this is happening is massively important.

12 *Excellent Journalists*

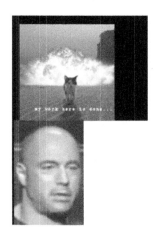 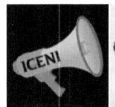 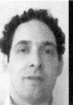 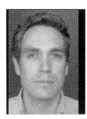 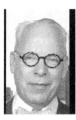 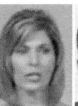

I honestly don't know whether No.'s 1 and 2 are journalists. I doubt it. They both know too much medical science. But I would never be able to live with myself if they did turn out to be journalists and I hadn't placed them on this very important list. My best guess would be cracker-jack PhD data analysts followed closely by M.D.- PhDs with the PhD part something requiring a lot of statistical analysis. I found only one clear error in three or four posts I read from these two, which is remarkable. There are two reasons I think these two are probably not medical doctors. 1) The error I found would not be made by a medical doctor as intelligent as these two, and, 2) one of the two recently made a very nice post about Climate Change.

I'm going to make a lot of posts about Climate Change when it comes back into favor, and I'm already at work on "Heroes and Villains: The Climate Change Book of Lists". I thought my interest in CO2's role in climate change was because I was a physics major and University physics instructor. This person could not be a medical doctor only. He understood the physics of climate change too well. A background in physics was more useful than medical knowledge in making my SARS-2 claims and explaining why expert-recommended policies could not work.

If the top two aren't journalists Alex and Freddie, take this category home.

1. **El Gato Malo**

This person is full of brilliant insights. He writes on Sub stack. I don't think he's an M.D. (too smart)

2. Spartacus

Trying to figure out the background of numbers 1 and 2 has been fun. I don't think Spartacus is a medical person. He mispronounces too many words on his "Spartacast". In written form, you'd never know. He's that good. He has a young voice. My best guess is he's between 30 and 35 years of age. Another Substacker.

3. Alex Berenson

Alex is so sharp. I don't understand why he doesn't see that the trial data show efficacy for ivermectin in prophylaxis and treatment .

4. Freddie Sayers

Freddie works for UnHerd which is supposed to be giving a forum, through interviews, to unheard ideas and the people who have them, thus the name. In this respect, he has failed me miserably as I have struggled since the beginning to get exposure. I made early, insightful and perfectly accurate posts. Facebook took them down within hours. I made 50 hours of videos, equally prescient, without flaw and full of insights that had not been seen or heard anywhere else. YouTube took some of them down within minutes. One of these had four views and two likes, one of which was mine! Nevertheless, I don't hold this against Freddie and the other interviewers who skipped over me. He's objective and plays a very good devil's advocate. Maybe when this book comes out?

4. Jeffrey Tucker
5. Sharyl Atkisson

6. Josh Rogin

Josh writes for the Washington Post and did some good work on the origin of the virus. He wrote about the "fox guarding the henhouse" aspects of the investigations by the Lancet, WHO, US Government, etc., having Peter Daszak leading the investigative team and so forth, which was helpful in understanding how those people who were actually there and were supposed to be experts couldn't figure out what I figured out in ten minutes and posted on Facebook in February 20, 2020, namely the proof that the virus was created in a lab.

8. Joe Rogan

Joe isn't a journalist in the traditional sense but he is a world-beater in the non-traditional one. I'm comfortable calling him a journalist because he's on the asking questions side of the interview. And he does tons of them. People trying to take him down from the air last year because of supposed misinformation spreading was ridiculous. Neil Young and Joni Mitchell were wrong for threatening to remove their music if he wasn't taken down. This arose out of long interviews Rogan did with Drs. Robert Malone and Peter McCullough who are very knowledgeable on the subject of COVID-19. The people supporting the corporate, pro vaccine, pro lockdowns, pro mask mandates, pro school closures Narrative want Rogan taken down. I never thought I'd see the day when Neil Young and Joni Mitchell would support the side they once abhorred, the corrupt Medical Industrial Complex.

Rogan is the last person you'd want taken down. He makes the occasional mistake when summarizing the facts but so would you or I if we weren't very knowledgeable doctors. He interviews both sides of the story and allows them to make their case. These singer songwriters wanted him taken down because of what his *guests* said. It's absurd. Should everyone who interviews Charlie Manson get taken off the air? And these two are far from Charles Manson. They are well-respected doctors; McCullough, primarily a clinician, Malone, a researcher.

I didn't agree with everything Drs. Malone and McCullough said, but I don't want Rogan taken off Spotify because of it. This guy is so humble and honest, if he remembers something differently than a guest, he asks his assistant to look it up on the spot. He's very intelligent and has a great feel for the questions the common man or woman want answered. He has a lot to be proud of but he doesn't come off as boastful in any way. A very talented guy with great values. You can tell when he talks about raising his children. Rogan is a breath of fresh air: humble, intelligent, masterful at what he does and loaded with integrity. We need more like him, especially now.

9. Jeremy Hammond

10. Kim Iverson

Kim was the best interviewer, analyst and personality on Rising. The way I understand her departure from the show, the producers/executives wouldn't let her interview Dr. Fauci the way she wanted to. So she left. Good on her.

11. Guy Gin

Reports from Japan. It's been very important to see how the Japanese customs affect the adoption of so many idiotic policies. And Guy Gin does it beautifully and bravely. He's been good at statistics too.

12.Alex Gutentag

Permanently suspended from Twitter on June 16, 2022, she was reinstated a day later due to public outcry. Described by Dr. Martin Kulldorff this way: "Her excellent journalism on the pandemic is grounded in science, basic principles of public health and deep compassion for fellow Americans."

12 Who Must Testify Under Oath re: Their Role in Thwarting Investigations into the Origin of the SARS-2 Virus

1. **Peter Daszak**
2. **Francis Collins**
3. **Anthony Fauci**
4. **Zheng Shi Li**
5. **Ralph Baric**
6. **Jeremy Farrar**
7. **James LeDuc**
8. **Kristian Andersen**
9. **Robert Garry**
10. **Ian Lipkin**
11. **Andrew Rambault**
12. **Edward C. Holmes**

32 Substakers, Patreon Posters, Bloggers, FB Posters Podcasters, Etc., Who Joined Forces To Mop the Floor With the "Experts".

What a job this team of people did! I can't rank you ladies and gentlemen. Each one of you contributed in your own way.

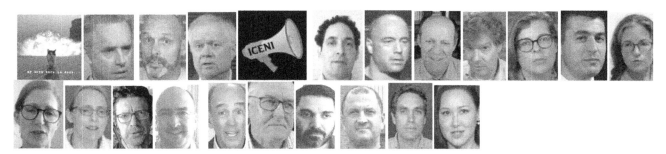

1. El Gato Malo
2. Jordan Peterson

Jordan isn't a COVID warrior per se but he belongs on this list because he has contributed so significantly to the war against free speech restrictions, postmodernism, and many other things germane to beating back the

3. Ivor Cummins
4. Chris Martenson, PhD

Very intelligent guy. I'd like to see him debate someone from the other side. By the way, many of the team of Substackers/podcasters, etc. listed here interview each other, which is fine. I haven't been able to break into this circuit yet but it wasn't for lack of trying. There's got to be something about me that is holding me back from being invited on these shows. Chris is one of the guys I wrote. I never heard back from him. Maybe in the future.

5. Spartacus
6. Alex Berenson
7. Joe Rogan
8. Steve Kirsch
9. Bret Weinstein, PhD

Bret's is one of the most interesting stories in this collection. It's like he was in the right place at the right time and parlayed it into enormous influence in a field he is not educated in. He was a professor at Evergreen College in Washington when he was the victim of threats by students during extended protests that got out of control with outrageous demands. It was a strange dynamic because, if I'm not mistaken, Bret is a progressive. I'm not sure how that mess got resolved.

Bret's speech is very measured, especially in interviews; no words are out of place. It's as considered as if someone had poured over it with pen and paper. Bret and his wife Heather have PhDs in Evolutionary Biology, so, through no fault of his own, he gets asked COVID-19 questions that are outside his field of expertise and to which he doesn't know the answer. In his early interviews, I noticed he was not willing to say, "I don't know" enough and he made a lot of mistakes. He's gotten much better. My opinion of him has improved as he has made this important transition. He has a very popular podcast as do many of the people on this list.

I recently heard he is catching flak from Sam Harris and others for his stance on early treatments and the mRNA vaccines. I don't understand this. To his detractors: If you think he's wrong about something, go on his show and debate him! Bret was on the top of his game in a Freddie Sayers interview I saw on YouTube recently. It was very interesting and Freddie, as always, asked great questions that got to the core of what Harris and the others are complaining about.

10. Heather Heying, PhD
10. Lex Fridman
10. Who is Robert Malone?
10. The Naked Emperor
10. Guy Gin
10. Arkmedic
10. Sage Hana
10. Matthew Crawford
10. Byram Bridle, PhD
10. Joomi
10. Jessica Rose, PhD
10. Larry Isaacs, M.D.
10. Tess Lawrie, MBBS, PhD
10. Dr. Clare Craig
10. Matthew B. Crawford
10. Eugyppius
10. Toby Rogers, PhD
10, Joseph Mercola, D.O.
10.John Campbell, PhD
10. Alexandros Marinos
10. Igor Chudov
10. Freddie Sayers
10. Kim Iverson

30 People I'd Like to Debate

1. **Anthony Fauci, M.D.** on the origin of the SARS-2 virus.
2. **Marty Makary, M.D.** on lockdowns (Dr. Makary was in favor of broad lockdowns to give time for hospitals to adjust. I have been strongly against them since the beginning and even warned against the death and destruction they would cause *before* they were put in place)
3. **Randi Weingarten**, on closing schools. (She pushed for them to be and stay closed.)
4. **Deborah Birx**, **M.D.** on Lockdowns.
5. **Kristian Andersen, PhD** on the origin of SARS-2. I say from a lab (humans were involved in creating parts of it), he says natural origins.
6. **Rochelle Walensky**, **M.D., MPH** on the justification for giving vaccines to six-month to five-year-old children (She endorsed the practice and actively promoted it.)

7. Barbara Ferrer, on closing public parks and beaches during the pandemic.

8. Joe Biden on vaccine mandates and requirements to vaccinate employees or fire them.

9. John Ioannidis, M.D. on whether generalized surgical mask use has non-negligible efficacy. He said he thought masks are "about 10% effective" at blocking transmission of the virus. I say they do not block viral transmission significantly.

10. Jonathan Reiner, M.D. on whether contact tracing is beneficial for an invisible respiratory virus that spreads by aerosols. (He kept asking for testing and tracing many months after the virus was "loose".)

11. Leana Wen, on whether 6 feet of physical distancing makes any sense.

12. Robert Redfield on whether surgical mask use is superior to a real vaccine with 70% effectiveness.

13. Tedros Adhanom Ghebreyesus on whether or not there was a group of people immune to SARS-2 before the virus arrived on our shores. (He said no one was immune. I say many people had immunity-in-place.)

14. Anthony Fauci, on whether gain of function research was conducted in Wuhan during the years 2014 − 2019.

15. Atul Guwande on whether COVID-19 mRNA vaccines confer better protection than getting and recovering from the disease. (He claims they do)

16. Albert Bourla, Stephan Bancel, Alex Gorsky, and Pascal Soriot on what is the best protein upon which to base the mRNA vaccines. They all made what would be considered by virtually all in the industry to be a very poor choice.

17. Barbara Ferrer on reintroducing indoor mask mandates in Los Angeles this fall.

18. Any University President, on the justification for requiring their students wear masks on campus this Fall, 2022; really at any time.

19. Jonathan Reiner on the need to vaccinate 60- 70- 90% plus of the population before herd immunity can be reached. (I proved we reached it on January 11, 2021 without a single person fully-vaccinated).

20. Francis Collins on the origin of the virus. He thinks it's a conspiracy theory that the vaccine was created in a lab.

21. Justin Trudeau on requiring airline passengers to get vaccinated before being allowed to board. He requires it even though the vaccines don't block transmission.

22. David Kessler, on authorizing the vaccine for six-month to five-year-olds. (He is in favor of it based on the trial data. I am not.)

23. Ashish Jha, on whether there have been any serious side effects from the vaccines and how many. He claims there have been none.

24. Leana Wen, M.D. on whether lockdowns were ever justified.

25. Deborah Birx, M.D. on whether or not lockdowns worked during the COVID-19 pandemic

26. Anyone who signed Peter Daszak's Lancet letter on the origin of the SARS-2 virus. (They all claim it arose naturally through an animal host and that claims it was made in a lab constitute a conspiracy theory

27. Anyone on the Stanford Medical School Faculty who signed the letter denouncing Scott Atlas on any subject brought up in the letter.

28. Dr. F. Perry Wilson on "Lockdowns: Did they 'flatten the curve' as promised?"

29. Leana Wen, M.D. on whether community masking can significantly reduce spread of a 100 nanometer virus transmitted by aerosols

30. **Dr. F. Perry Wilson** on whether the vaccines were beneficial.

Chapter 2 (Places)

10 *Universities That Displayed COVID-Science Illiteracy*

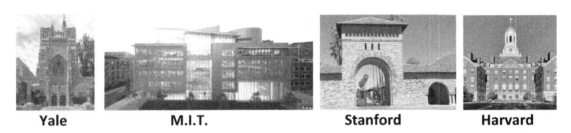

Yale   M.I.T.   Stanford   Harvard

1. Yale

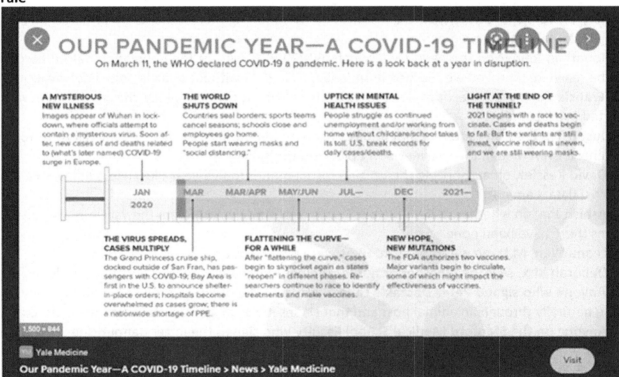

Yale has embarrassed itself by pumping out reams of idiotic information.

Just about everything on Yale's timeline is incorrect. Note that it's a "look back". It's not a prediction. There is no excuse for being this inaccurate. Yale medicine simply could not interpret graphs correctly and they were incorrect in assigning the reasons for the peaks and troughs. Going through from left to right, "A MYSTERIOUS NEW ILLNESS", January, 2020. We knew it was a coronavirus from the beginning. (WHO Director General Tedros was not telling the truth when he said it "is a new virus and nobody has immunity to it.") We also knew it was in Italy before November 21, 2019, because it was isolated from a little boy's throat in Milan on that date. It had been circulating around for at least two months and nobody noticed.

The timeline says "soon after January, 2020, new cases and deaths surge in Europe". That's not correct. It wasn't until the last days of February, that cases started shooting up in Italy. Precise dates are very important if we are to get to the bottom of this fraud. There were only 2.43 cases per day in Italy on February 21, 2020. They shot up from that point until March 26 when they reached their peak at 5,650 confirmed cases per day. Contrary to popular belief, the U.S. was only two weeks behind Italy, with the northeast wave reaching its peak on April 10 at 31,979 cases per day.

Recall that it was on March 8 for me and near that date for Dr. Michael Levitt when we determined independently, using data from the Diamond Princess Cruise Ship outbreak, that the infection fatality rate (IFR) was actually .1%, (my number. I think Dr. Levitt's was a little higher) thereby showing the "experts" had it 40 times too high at 4%. Recall also that it was March 24, 2020, when the CDC changed the guidelines for reporting COVID-19 fatalities from one that was in existence for 17 years, into one that included any death within 28 days of a positive PCR test, leading to wildly exaggerated death counts which included "because of" and "with" COVID (and sometimes neither of these because the PCR test at 40 cycles produced so many false positive results.) It's quite possible that when the powers behind all of this realized they weren't going to get death counts high enough to scare people into the manipulations they wanted to effectuate, they changed the Guidelines to make the pandemic look much worse than it was.

THE VIRUS SPREADS, CASES MULTIPLY This was certainly true but except for a very few exceptions, hospitals weren't "overwhelmed". This was the time when hospital nurses were posting crazy line dancing videos due to not having enough to do. (If you don't remember this, take a look at this video: https://www.youtube.com/watch?v=yhUAJRYA3bk)

THE WORLD SHUTS DOWN The world didn't shut down because of the virus. The politicians shut the world down for other reasons. They used the virus as an excuse.

FLATTENING THE CURVE- FOR A WHILE There was no flattening of any curves at any time in any country. Yale thinks the trough between the bumps in the Northeast and South was due to flattening the curve. That is beyond idiotic. Then they blame the second "bump" (which was the first wave hitting the South) on states reopening. No, it was just the first wave in a different climate zone.

LIGHT AT THE END OF THE TUNNEL? Cases and deaths did begin to fall but vaccines had nothing to do with it. We reached herd immunity to the Wuhan strain on January 11, 2021. We did so without a single person being fully-vaccinated.

95

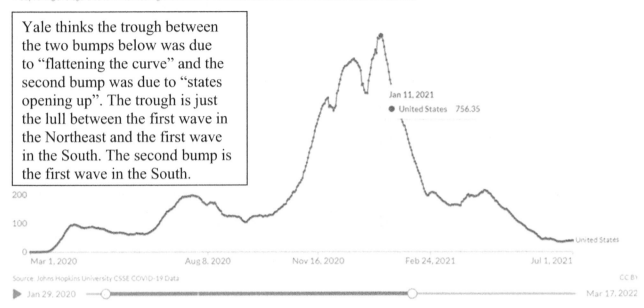

Yale thinks the trough between the two bumps below was due to "flattening the curve" and the second bump was due to "states opening up". The trough is just the lull between the first wave in the Northeast and the first wave in the South. The second bump is the first wave in the South.

Jan 11, 2021
● United States   756.35

200

100

0

Mar 1, 2020   Aug 8, 2020   Nov 16, 2020   Feb 24, 2021   Jul 1, 2021

United States

Source: Johns Hopkins University CSSE COVID-19 Data   CC BY

▶ Jan 29, 2020 ─────○──────────────────────────────○────────────── Mar 17, 2022

2. M.I.T.

M.I.T. wasn't more incorrect than any of the other Universities on this list. They get ranked second because they should have known better. M.I.T., perhaps more than any other University in the world, is "science incorporated". It has an aura about it that everyone feels when they visit the place. Even after you've been there a few years, you walk down the infinite corridor and catch the eye of another student- "Can you believe we're here?" The place is wall-to-wall magic.

We needed M.I.T. to take the lead on this but they failed. There's an easy explanation for it and it's not very becoming. MIT didn't want to lose the enormous funding they receive every year from the NIH and other government bodies; some of it, I'm sure, from the hand of Anthony Fauci. So they accepted the status quo.

Yes, it's shameful. I love MIT and I'll be eternally grateful to them for taking a chance on a naive kid who hadn't taken physics or calculus in high school, but I can't give MIT a pass on this. That same naïve kid figured out the entire thing from start to finish by reasoning from first principles while MIT, who has been ranked the #1 University in the world for 12 straight years by the QS World University Rankings, couldn't even figure out that lockdowns were a bad idea.

The sad truth is that M.I.T. has gone woke.

A lot of us who graduated more than 20 years ago didn't realize how bad it had gotten at MIT. But then we started to notice stories in the news like the firing of John Moloney, MIT's Catholic chaplain, for weighing in on the death of George Floyd and the protests that followed, in a way that "contradicted the Institute's values" and was "deeply disturbing" according to Suzy Nelson, vice president and dean for student life. What had this priest written in an email to the Tech Catholic Community that was "deeply disturbing"?

Moloney wrote that while Floyd should not have been killed by a police officer, Floyd's killing was not necessarily "an act of racism", adding that "people have claimed that racism" is a "major problem in police forces. I don't think we know that." He wrote that the police officer had "acted wrongly" and that "it is right that he has been arrested and will be prosecuted."Moloney also wrote that Floyd "had not lived a virtuous life," stating that Floyd had committed sins, "but we do not kill such people" and instead "root for sinners to change their lives and convert to the Gospel."

Suzy Nelson, vice president and dean for student life, wrote in an email to student and faculty leaders that the Bias Response Team had received reports about Moloney's email. She wrote that Moloney's message "contradicted the Institute's values" and "was deeply disturbing." That was her opinion and she's free to have it, speak it and write it. She should have, however, explained *in what way* it "contradicted the Institute's values" and "was deeply disturbing". She never did, of course, which is typical of woke attacks on speech they don't agree with. This is true with COVID as well, where we can't get anyone supporting the Narrative to debate anything. We're heading down a very dark path when scientific matters of great importance cannot be debated freely.

I can tell you as a surgeon with 34 years behind the walls including three residencies that Moloney was incorrect in assuming Floyd was killed by the police officer in question, Derek Chauvin. I've made videos:

https://www.youtube.com/watch?v=h-v_AsN9oeg&t=215s and

https://www.youtube.com/watch?v=IvXbsaK5EWs&t=12s showing why the expert witnesses were wrong on many critical aspects of the case. There isn't anything else Moloney said that was incorrect.

1. "The killing was not necessarily an act of racism". Correct. The prosecuting attorney didn't even bring in racism as a motivating factor.

2. "People have claimed that racism is a major problem in police forces. I don't think we know that". Correct. If anything, studies show the opposite- that police are reluctant to use force against blacks or to pull them over for traffic violations for fear of being labeled racist. If you are unaware of this, watch this video: https://www.youtube.com/watch?v=IPwAVecR3DI. Think about the assertion by the (black) Harvard data analyst that the myth that police treat blacks unfairly is hurting blacks. It's true and it's a disgrace.

3. Moloney wrote that the police officer had "acted wrongly" and that "it is right that he has been arrested and will be prosecuted." Officer Chauvin definitely "acted wrongly" in some ways. For one, he didn't try to revive Floyd when he went unconscious. But he didn't cause his death. Someone Chauvin's size plus equipment can't compress someone's trachea, the size of Floyd, by putting his knee on the back of Floyd's neck. It cannot be done and the autopsy results confirmed it. The trachea and surrounding structures were not disturbed in any way. Adjacent muscles showed no signs of trauma. There was plenty of evidence on the video tape too, as hard as it was to watch. You'll fight someone who is choking you. Floyd didn't do that. He just drifted away as if he was falling asleep, like you do under the influence of a narcotic overdose. The video demonstrated this clearly. Finally, until he went unconscious, Floyd talked the entire time Chauvin was on him. You cannot talk when your trachea is blocked to air passage. Chauvin was innocent of what they charged him with while possibly being guilty of something else.

4. Was it that he wrote that Floyd "had not lived a virtuous life" and that he had "committed sins"? Was that the part of Moloney's message that Suzi Nelson found "deeply disturbing"? Floyd did hold a gun to a pregnant woman's belly while his accomplices broke into her home and robbed it. Call me crazy but I'd say that qualifies as a sin. I'd also say that being in and out of prison for armed robbery in addition to other serious offences is not consistent with living a virtuous life.

According to Nelson's email, all MIT chaplains sign the Office of Religious, Spiritual, and Ethical Life's "Relationship with Affiliated Organizations and Representatives" agreement, which states that chaplains should demonstrate "respect for the dignity and worth of all people and a sensitivity to the beliefs and cultural commitments of others" and that "actions or statements that diminish the value of individuals or groups of people are prohibited." Nelson wrote that Moloney's email did not "live up to these expectations." You could also make a case that Ms. Nelson is not showing respect for the dignity and worth of the pregnant woman and her unborn child at whom Mr. Floyd pointed the gun while his accomplices robbed her house.

M.I.T.'s next blunder was in canceling the speech of geophysicist Dorian Abbot's scheduled lecture on Climate Change because of his opinion that college admissions should be merit-based and not be driven by diversity, equity and inclusion (DEI). Abbot expressed this opinion in a Newsweek article earlier that Fall and it sent the heads of woke academia spinning.

Abbot is all for recruiting minorities. He just thinks it's wrong to focus on DEI in college admissions, saying it "violates the ethical and legal principle of equal treatment" and "entails treating people as members of a group rather than as individuals, repeating the mistake that made possible the atrocities of the 20th century." It's hardly a far right, radical position. The state of California – California, mind you- opposes race-based college admissions, employment, and contracting. Abbot went on to elucidate his position by proposing an admissions based on "Merit, Fairness, and Equality (MFE), whereby university applicants are treated as individuals and evaluated through a rigorous and unbiased process based on their merit and qualifications alone." This would also mean ending legacy and athletic admissions advantages, which generally favor white applicants.

M.I.T. and Caltech famously do not consider legacy or athletic prowess, per se, in admissions and they're on the right side of that argument when you're talking about our most elite academic institutions. That is not to say M.I.T. doesn't see value in athletics. Until just a few years ago, M.I.T. fielded more teams at the varsity level than any university in America.

The prestigious John Carlson Lecture which Dr. Abbot was disinvited to give, falls within the department of Earth, Atmospheric and Planetary Sciences, and it was Department Chairman, Robert Van der Hilst, who caved to the Twitter mob and canceled the lecture. He's still trying to justify it. Something about the lecture being open to the public, including high school students, and not wanting to offend them... Yeah, so let's deprive those students of the chance to visit M.I.T. and see a great lecture because some grad students (and perhaps the Chairman himself) disagreed with the speaker on merit-based vs. race-based admissions policies and of course the bigger question of whether society should consider people as individuals or as members of this group or that. Abbot's perfectly reasonable stance on race-based admissions had nothing to do with the subject of his lecture, "New Developments in Climate Science". Is M.I.T. going to be responsible for every political position of every speaker it invites from now on?

A Princeton University professor was on the phone as soon as he heard, inviting Professor Abbot down to New Jersey, on the same date, to deliver the lecture. Abbot accepted. Princeton: 1, M.I.T.: 0

Raphael Reif will step down this year as M.I.T.'s President and it's time for M.I.T. to reject the woke policies, ethos and culture it had fallen into over the last couple of decades under Dr. Reif's leadership. M.I.T. needs to find its way back to the political neutrality it prided itself on before Reif took office.

3. Stanford

One hundred six scientists and medical doctors associated with the Stanford School of Medicine endorsed mask use by the general public despite decades of research showing it does not change transmission significantly. They did so by signing the letter denouncing Dr. Scott Atlas, a person who understood the medical science behind COVID-19 better than any of the 106. He also knew the epidemiology and public health issues better than them, even though many of them were epidemiologists and public health specialists. Others ran studies that showed they did not understand that antibodies have a finite half-life, that immunity-in-place exists due to cross-reactivity, and that patients who no longer have antibodies circulating in their blood may still be protected from getting a disease due to clonal expansion and memory of B and T cells. This is all very basic, freshman-level knowledge they should have had complete command over. This is Stanford University, remember, not Podunk Central

4. Harvard

Would you expect anything different from Harvard? Lots and lots of parents contacted the registrar asking for partial reimbursement of tuition because the classes were being taught over the internet. What happened? Well let's put it this way, The infamous Jeffrey Epstein visited M.I.T. and Harvard frequently and made several major donations to both schools, starting in the late 1990s.

M.I.T. gave all the money back and embarked on an investigation, creating a big brouhaha. As for Harvard, here is how they handled the controversy: "Mr. Epstein's gift is funding important research using mathematics to study areas such as evolutionary theory, viruses, and cancers," a university spokesman said. "The University is not considering returning this gift." Do you think Harvard is going to reimburse parents over the inferior education their children received because of pandemic orders from on high? No chance.

5. Princeton

6. University of Chicago

7. Amherst

8. NYU

NYU requires that all eligible students receive a booster by July 15, 2022. Requiring any of the Vaccines, now that the deadly side effects are known, is playing Russian Roulette with the student body. Pfizer and the other vaccine makers may be immune to problems arising out of their use, but Universities and employers who are requiring these horrible injections are not. Imagine the lawsuits...

9. UCSF College of Medicine

I am shocked to discover so many instructors at this once-prestigious medical school still don't understand the basic and clinical science surrounding COVID-19 and the measures undertaken to combat it. Yet another example is Bryn Boslett, M.D. who states in "COVID-19 Vaccine Fact vs. Fiction: An Expert Weighs in on Common Fears" that, "This is not a live virus vaccine, and the mRNA is likely going to stay right in the arm where it's injected and get taken up by the cells there. The mRNA is quickly degraded by the body after it does its job." Both of these sentences relate to vitally-important matters and are incorrect.

10. Georgetown

Georgetown is still requiring masks in the fall term of 2022. Here are the Guidelines: "Masks are still required in indoor instructional settings such as classrooms and teaching laboratories on the Main and Medical Center Campuses. This applies to organized classes but not to informal gatherings (e.g. in libraries and study spaces)." This makes no sense at all. If someone was infected, they would be blowing out most of the virus through the sides of their mask right into the sides of the mask being worn by the person sitting next to them, looking in the same direction (as in a class when both are looking at the lecturer). That is, if masks worked, which they don't. The Guidelines go on to say, "Individuals in, or recently released from, quarantine or isolation, must wear a mask for the full 10 days from the date of exposure or infection."

All of these guidelines are idiotic. Masks don't do anything significant to reduce the spread of the virus and they do a lot of harm.

10 Institutions That Got More Respect Than They Deserved

1. The US FDA

This place deserves almost no respect. It has gotten so corrupt and/or incompetent, it's mindboggling. Look at the official reason they gave for taking away the EUA for hydroxychloroquine (HCQ). Note that my disgust with the FDA has nothing to do with whether or not HCQ works. My disgust arises out of the FDA's inability to measure the proper endpoints for the cohort claimed to benefit from the treatment. (The underlining is mine) "June 15, 2020 Update: Based on ongoing analysis and emerging scientific data, FDA has revoked the emergency use authorization (EUA) to use HCQ and chloroquine to treat COVID-19 in certain hospitalized patients when a clinical trial is unavailable or participation is not feasible. We made this determination based on recent results from a large, randomized clinical trial in hospitalized patients that found these medicines showed no benefit for decreasing the likelihood of death or speeding recovery. This outcome was consistent with other new data, including those showing the suggested dosing for these medicines are unlikely to kill or inhibit the virus that causes COVID-19. As a result, we determined that the legal criteria for the EUA are no longer met."

Just to make it crystal clear for those who do not understand why I underlined the two phrases: The first underline of the words "hospitalized patients": The cohort claimed to benefit by the use of HCQ did not consist of hospitalized patients. It was made up of high-risk ambulatory outpatients who were able to start treatment shortly after first noticing symptoms. The second: No one claimed HCQ worked because of its ability to "kill or inhibit the virus". HCQ has many modes of action, including its ability to modulate the immune response. This is one of the main reasons why it is used for Rheumatoid Arthritis. So the FDA was so incompetent, they measured the wrong endpoint for the wrong cohort (or they were told to design the study so that it would fail to show efficacy).

HCQ is over the counter in many, many countries. Imagine how family members of the deceased feel about the FDA removing the EUA for a cheap and very safe alternative that would have saved their loved one's life and that the FDA did this because of incompetence or corruption. Imagine, also, how they feel about YouTube for taking down videos claiming that HCQ is safe (which it clearly is), for the same reasons- incompetence and/or corruption. And there were many other early treatments that were not considered by the FDA for EUA, treatments that showed clear efficacy against SARS-2 infection, hospitalization, and death.

This is another example of trying to determine whether stupidity and incompetence caused the FDA Advisory committee to take away HCQ's EUA or was it that the vaccine makers knew they couldn't get an EUA for their vaccines if there was an effective alternate treatment available, and put pressure on committee members making the decision at the FDA. The overwhelming likelihood is that people at the FDA fell victim to pressure –monetary perhaps- to keep these medicines off the market. Basically, they were willing to let people die for money.

2. The US NIAID

Dr. Anthony Fauci has been running this subsidiary of the NIH since 1984. His performance at the NIAID as an AIDS epidemic combatant, first as a researcher and then as Director, pushing AZT when safer medicines were effective, damaged his and the Institution's reputations profoundly. His performance ginning up uncalled-for fear in subsequent outbreaks did his reputation nothing of benefit for scientists in the know. For the last 2 ½ years he has continued much of the same, supporting, even pushing the use of dangerous, ineffective, and expensive treatments on the public while clearly not understanding the science behind the latest viral epidemic/pandemic. All the way from the gain of function research that was moved to China with his assistance, to the present day, Dr. Fauci has claimed that there is no reason people should be walking around wearing masks. Then he said he lied about that to prevent the public from taking the supply of surgical masks from healthcare workers. He then recommended cloth masks and said they were effective. This is inconsistent. He could have recommended cloth masks early on if he was worried about the public taking all of the surgical masks; that is if he was telling us the truth about why he said they don't work. This is enough to tell me that he was lying about the reason for saying "masks don't work". The only thing that makes sense is that the reason for originally saying there's no reason for people to go around wearing masks" is because he knew over many years of studies, that masks don't work. Then someone gave him a memo telling him to push masks because someone wanted the people to wear them. You will recall, in October of 2020, he was trying to get people to wear two masks. The mask is a perfect symbol for taking away what makes an individual, an individual, their ability to express their unique thoughts and opinions.

3. The US NIH

Here is just a partial list of what the NIH has done in the last handful of years:

1. They funded, with US AID Peter Daszak's Eco Health Alliance (EHA) gain of function research at the Wuhan Institute of Virology during the time there was a moratorium placed on this activity. This funding resulted in the creation of SARS-2, a virus that has killed millions of people and with the help of some very stupid government officials, some of which are employed by the NIH, shut down the world for two years. This will result in more than 100 million more deaths.

2. Tried to cover up their funding and involvement in the activities in Wuhan by attacking the reputations of people who suggested the virus may have been created in a lab.

3. Failed to engage P3CO analysis of the EHA program in Wuhan when it was clearly indicated.

4. Failed to disclose neither the members of their P3CO advisory committee nor their findings and recommendations.

5. Received royalty kickbacks from pharmaceutical companies amounting to $350 million, a blatant conflict of interest.

6. From Director Francis Collins, the claim that masks prevent the spread of SARS-2.

7. Per Director Francis Collins's request, attempted a "devastating takedown" of the Great Barrington Declaration authored by three "fringe epidemiologists".

This partial list has destroyed all trust in and respect for the once-cherished Institution.

4. The US CDC
5. The WHO
6. Johns Hopkins University School of Medicine
7. Stanford University School of Medicine

8. The American Academy of Pediatrics
Who in their right mind could respect an organization that endorses masking two-year-olds
   9.   **Yale University**
   10.   **All U.S.Specialty Boards.**

13 Institutions/Organizations Who's Reputations Took the Biggest Hit

1. The US CDC
2. The US NIH
3. The US FDA
How was the FDA not ranked #1 since they are the ones who approved the worthless and harmful vaccines AND they were the ones who demanded the trial data be hidden for 75 years, the trial upon which those approvals were based? It depends on how far an institution had to fall. The FDA had almost completely destroyed their reputation before COVID-19 started. They fell quickly but they didn't have as far to fall as did the CDC and NIH. The CDC had more goodwill to begin with. They lost it all too, as did the NIH.

4. Johns Hopkins University School of Medicine
Hopkins is a medical school that used to have a stellar reputation. But they completely botched the daily new case and death counts for the U.S. and worldwide by a factor of as much as 17.2. They also put out tons of false messaging about the efficacy of mask use by the general public. Here's a quote from Hopkinsmedicine.org: "Both influenza and SARS-2 can be PREVENTED by mask-wearing, frequent and thorough hand-washing, coughing into the crook of your elbow, staying home when sick, and limiting contact with people who are infected."

5. The American Academy of Pediatrics
These people claimed that mask mandates worked from age two years and above. Well-designed studies were then done in Finland that proved them 100% wrong of course. But when an organization like the AAP makes a statement like that, even if it has been proved false, someone like the Mayor of New York City can use it to justify mask mandates in toddlers and preschoolers, which is exactly what he did. This results in poor dental health and stunted speaking and language skills in these children.

6. Imperial College, London
7. The Lancet
   From the papers they had to retract to the Daszak "Lab Origin is a conspiracy theory" letter they printed, this once-prestigious medical journal will need a long time to regain its reputation.

8. The New England Journal of Medicine
   As was the case with the Lancet, recalling papers severely damaged the reputation of perhaps the most prestigious medical journal in the world. It doesn't help to have laymen writing articles with the words 'Pandemic of the Century' in the title.

9. Stanford University School of Medicine
10. S.A.G.E.
11. The EMA
12. The Massachusetts General Hospital
Ordinarily, an Institution that sends one of their own to do their duty as NIH, FDA, or CDC Director would gain notoriety and position in the world. Not this time for this Institution. A number of their doctors made significant errors during Covid-19. Rochelle Walensky has not lived up to what people expected of her.

She's had trouble at times, understanding the numbers coming out of the trials. She was very late, along with Dr. Fauci in realizing that the vaccine was not capable of blocking transmission of the virus. Also, Dr. Walensky presided over an organization that withheld data, refused to debate the policies many people took issue with and pushed vaccines in small children and babies whose approval was not justified by the trial data.

13. Yale School of Medicine

Yale has a doctor who is quite talented in the speaking department, who presents on various topics. He is so wrong about some of them, you can see it on his face. His presentation on lockdowns reminds one of a forced confession from an underground, rat-infested jail cell during the Iran hostage crisis. When I see Dr. F. Perry Wilson next time, I'm going to ask him when he got out.

Dr. Wilson said, "Vaccines have performed better in this pandemic than we had any right to hope for". Really? What data are you looking at, doctor? and…"Well, the idea is that we need to slow the spread of the disease and the number one thing that we've focused on for much of this pandemic has been vaccination which has been incredibly successful." –Dr. F. Perry Wilson on CNN, January 14, 2022.

Really, Dr. Wilson? Weren't masks and social distancing and lockdowns and school closures invoked to slow the spread? None of them worked but that was the ostensible reason for putting them in place, right? But you say the number one thing we've focused on to slow the spread is vaccination and it has been "incredibly successful? That is not even close to the truth. They haven't been even minimally successful.. In fact, they've done enormous harm.

This particular CNN interview was almost exactly one year after I showed the vaccines were not blocking spread. When Dr. Wilson said this on national TV, the virus had already spread like wildfire through the vaccinated population. Even Drs. Fauci and Walensky were admitting the vaccines didn't block transmission by then.

Dr. Wilson also showed a ludicrous graph from a study in Nature claiming that predicted deaths were higher than after lockdowns were put in place. It's pictured below. Predicted deaths were higher because the models were so bad (see "1 Inaccurate Modeler") It had nothing to do with lockdowns. Sweden's predicted deaths were more than seven times higher than what came to pass (and that's including "with" COVID) and they didn't use lockdowns! It was utterly preposterous for Dr. Wilson to use wildly inaccurate predictions to compare against reality and conclude that some intervention accounted for the difference. The truth is that lockdowns didn't cause any significant reductions in deaths in any country at any time. They actually increased deaths slightly, in-and-of-themselves. I have explained why and shown that the data confirms it. When you put the European countries side by side on the same screen, you can't tell which one didn't use lockdowns. That's just one of 1000 graphs I could show you that say lockdowns didn't do anything beneficial. They did, however, cause enormous death and destruction through collateral damage. Even the WHO predicts 140 million people will starve to death because of supply chain disruptions. Add to that the deaths from people not getting cancer screenings and the deaths now resulting from moratoria placed on all but emergency surgery and you can see that lockdowns lead to giant multiples of the six million deaths "because of" and "with", COVID.

"Predicted deaths were higher than those observed once lockdowns were put in place? " No, they weren't (meaning it was due to bad predictions, not anything lockdowns did).

14. UCSF Medical School

This Medical School used to be one of the 15 finest in the US. But during the pandemic, all kinds of bizarre and idiotic recommendations came out of their faculty in addition to gross data misinterpretation. Here's an example from Monica Gandhi, M.D., an internal medicine professor there: "While I'm almost positive that vaccination is going to take away transmission, if you had a little viral RNA in your nose, we would never want a vaccinated person to pass that on to an unvaccinated person. So, mask around the unvaccinated until they are vaccinated too." Wow. She thinks wearing a mask by a vaccinated person will protect an unvaccinated person. She is also "almost positive that vaccination is going to take away transmission." No and No. It's not unimportant either. People hear this kind of nonsense and they think the vaccine blocks transmission. They also think wearing a mask protects the unvaccinated from the vaccinated. Then they go out and engage in risky behavior with the vulnerable. Plus, how can you tell who is vaccinated and who is not? Are you going to go around asking everyone in a restaurant? In the mall or in church?

15. The University of Washington They took people off of the transplant list for refusing to be vaccinated. When you do something like this, especially to children, you have done nothing less than declared war on civilized society.

Chapter 3 (Things)

9 Most Important Slides of the Pandemic

1.

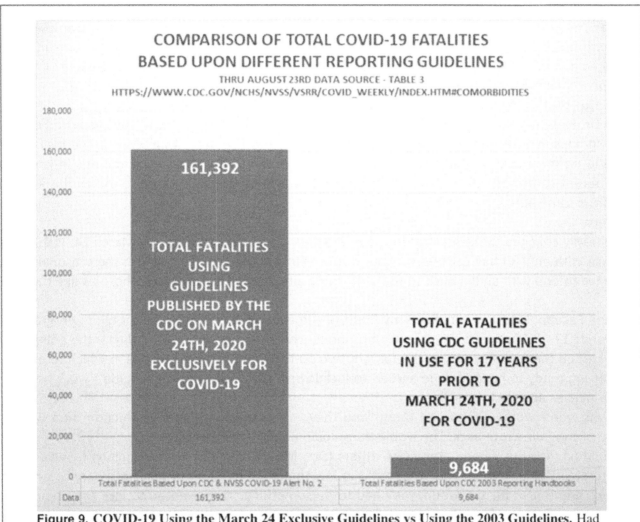

Figure 9. COVID-19 Using the March 24 Exclusive Guidelines vs Using the 2003 Guidelines. Had the CDC used the 2003 guidelines, the total **COVID-19** be approximately 16.7 times lower than is currently being reported. [1][30][State & Territory Health Departments]

Did you know that the Guidelines for reporting COVID-19 fatalities were changed by the CDC on March 24, 2020? The previous Guidelines had been in place for 17 years. As you can see from the bar-graph above, 161,392 COVID-19 fatalities were recorded through August 23, 2020. Had the CDC used the Guidelines that had been in place since 2003, only 9,684.Would have been recorded.

What is shocking is that there are very few people who know about this. The powers that be definitely did not want the public at large to know that these guidelines had been changed.

If I was a Senator in charge of a committee whose job it was to get to the bottom of why we shut down the world and caused death and destruction on a biblical scale over a virus that was less deadly than the seasonal flu for all but the very old, I'd call everyone in who had any say in changing the guidelines into something far less useful and far more vulnerable to exploitation by bad actors. Remember, for all but the very old, the original, Wuhan strain infection fatality rate (IFR) for COVID-19 was less than that of the seasonal flu. For working age and younger, it was even less than that! The guidelines were changed to include falling off of ladders, homicides, accidental poisonings, motor vehicle accidents, suicide and many others, or, as The Public Health Director of Illinois, Dr. Ezike, put it, "even if you died of a clear alternate cause of death but you had COVID at the same time, it's still listed as a COVID death. That means that everyone listed as a COVID death, it doesn't mean that was the *cause* of death but that they had COVID *at the time of death*. I hope that's helpful."

Yes, Dr. Ezike, that's very helpful.

When I saw Dr. Ezike say this for the first time, I lowered myself into a chair slowly, my eyes fixed on the screen, as I spoke softly, the way you do when you're speaking to yourself, "Murderers". The logic went through me in no more than a split second like the way a card counter bypasses arithmetic in knowing totals for different combinations of cards. He can and will use arithmetic if pressed to explain his actions and I will do the same here.

"Murderers."

They arbitrarily changed the guidelines for how fatalities were to be counted on March 24, 2020. This took a disease with an IFR I had calculated three weeks before to be less than that of the seasonal flu at .1% for all ages to one with an IFR back to the 3-4% originally claimed by various authorities like the CDC and WHO.

I had made Facebook posts to publicize my findings and even written four major network program TV hosts on March 17, 2020, two days after Trump announced that we would be, reluctantly, going into lockdowns. I asked those hosts- two on the far left, two on the right- for five minutes in which to explain what was getting ready to happen if we agreed to lockdowns. I knew lockdowns wouldn't work because of my first principles approach to problems.

"Lockdowns won't work", I informed them "and they will cause death and destruction on a Biblical scale". None of the four wrote back. The whole thing could have been averted.

I'm speculating now but when I and a few others (Drs. Mike Levitt and John Ioannidis) revealed that the infection fatality rate (IFR) for this virus was too low to induce the kind of fear necessary to be used for someone's grand plan for the world, they had to do something. They wanted to lock the population down and cover their mouths. Knowing that the public would never have accepted losing their livelihoods, life savings, medical insurance, etc.- everything that comes with losing their jobs-for a disease that was only worse than the flu in people beyond retirement age, they had to do something. That something turned out to be very simple. They just changed the guidelines.

The original IFR of 4% was faulty due to a too-low denominator in the equation that defines it:

IFR = # of deaths/ # of people infected

When you reduce the denominator in a quotient, the quotient increases. The denominator being used was less than reality because they were not counting those infected who did not exhibit symptoms. It's a very obvious form of selection bias. When that jig was up, they went after the numerator. They increased the number of deaths by more than an order of magnitude (more than 10x) by simply changing the guidelines. This made the IFR go from its actual value of .1%, up-up-up to a value that frightened everyone into shutting down the world over something that was no more than slightly worse than an average flu season.

Nothing actually changed, of course. We only changed the way we *recorded* it. The CDC purposefully reported a lie about the number of people who were actually dying from this disease. They weren't called out on it by the hospitals who knew different because the hospitals were profiting wildly as a result of the fraud. Our government was bribing them to keep their mouths shut. An economic study revealed that the hospitals brought in more than $50,000 per COVID patient, $50,000 of YOUR US taxpayer money. The actual number in the study was $100,000 but that included incentives for vaccinating employees and a few other things.

Many trained people didn't understand how the infection fatality rate was being manipulated, including medical doctors, epidemiologists, PhDs in immunology and virology, and people with Masters Degrees in public health. Many made videos and posts that were filled with incorrect information. Others appeared as guest experts on network TV supporting the fear narrative. Most of these people have disappeared now, knowing they did a terrible disservice to humankind, actually contributing to the loss of innocent lives. Some have stayed in the public eye, promoting the perpetuation of harmful non-pharmaceutical interventions At last, we are beginning to see some members of the public calling them out for it. They are listed later in this book

In summary, had the guidelines not been changed, we would have counted far fewer deaths all along. The factor by which deaths were exaggerated (16.7) on August 23, 2020, varied only slightly once mass testing was firmly in place. Mass testing with the terribly-flawed PCR test provided the perpetrators even more opportunities to fudge the figures.

Using the same factor of 16.7 tells us that instead of passing the one million mark three seasons into the pandemic on May 17, 2022, we would have passed the modest mark of 59,880 fatalities due to the SARS-2 coronavirus. This comes to a little less than 30,000 deaths per year, on par with the seasonal flu. Other analyses show about double that figure but the actual number of deaths was nowhere near one million on May 17, 2022. My best guess is that there were about 150,000 deaths at that point, implying that the actual deaths due to COVID-19 were about 15% of what we were told. (Please see Most important slide #7 below)

You can see why this simple bar graph tops the list. The incredibly destructive lockdowns, ineffective mask mandates, school closures that will shorten the lives of affected children, the worsening disaster that was born out of the supposed need to develop a vaccine in the midst of an ongoing pandemic- all of this and more- would have been avoided if someone hadn't changed the guidelines for assigning cause of death.

2.

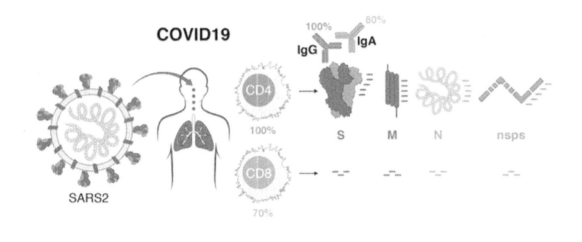

Before I discovered the bar graph ranked #1 above, the most important slide of the pandemic by a very significant margin was that which now takes the number 2 spot. I used this schematic to confirm why my early March suspicions were correct as to the reason why some Diamond Princess passengers did not come down with the virus despite being packed in like sardines with others that did. They had "immunity-in-place" a term I coined to describe their protection from infection arising out of cross reactivity with other coronaviruses with which they had come into contact. Likewise, this was the reason some nursing home patients were not affected by a horrible breakout in some facilities where several residents not only got the infection, but died from it. I also used this pair of diagrams in my proof that we reached herd immunity for the wild type on January 11, 2021 without a single person achieving the benefit of being fully vaccinated, and third, I used it, along with data from Israel, to confirm my suspicions from before the vaccines were released to the public, that the mRNA vaccines were incapable of blocking transmission of the virus. I proved this by assuming the vaccines were blocking transmission and deriving a contradiction.

These three observations are among the four or five most important insights of the entire pandemic with their implications regarding the need for mass vaccination, despite being unrecognized by everyone else at the time.

YouTube didn't do the world any favors by taking down, within minutes of its posting, my video explaining how we reached herd immunity for the original Wuhan strain without a single person being fully vaccinated against it. Millions of people were told or forced to get the vaccine in order to help us, as a society, reach herd immunity. That was completely incorrect and probably the first or second most egregious public health policy decision in history, the most other being lockdowns. Which one wins out between these two will depend on how the vaccine debacle we are living through now, pans out. At least 150 million people will die from collateral damage caused by the lockdowns. The vaccine disaster could lead to many more deaths. We do not know at present.

This schematic, taken from a study by Sette, Crotty et al, (Sette, 2020) proved WHO Director Tedros Adhanom Ghebreyesus wrong when he said, "COVID-19 is a new virus and nobody has immunity to it." This was a most reckless and irresponsible thing to say. First, the WHO Director's statement was 100% incorrect. Second, it steered people away from the proper course of action when they were considering whether or not to get vaccinated. ALL people considering this should have had themselves checked to see if they had immunity-in-place. Think of the hundreds of thousands of people and counting who died because they got the vaccine when they were already protected.

Recall that this was at a time when Fauci and the TV doctors were telling us on a daily basis that, 1) only 10% of the US population had been exposed to the virus based on studies from places like Stanford University, 2) that the vaccine was going to confer greater immunity than getting and recovering from the disease, and 3) that 60 – 70% , later increased to 90% and then 98% of the population needed to be vaccinated for us to reach herd immunity.

I proved that we reached herd immunity without a single *person* being fully vaccinated. This discovery would have thrown the entire Narrative on its ear and destroyed the notion that we needed mass vaccination to end the pandemic. The truth is that we not only did not need mass vaccination to get through this pandemic, doing so caused the pandemic to continue due to the production of new variants the emergence of which depend on vaccination. The production of non-neutralizing antibodies toward an actively replicating virus in the midst of a pandemic puts selective pressure on the emergence of new strains, benefitting proliferation of those strains so selected. This is one of the ways Operation Warp Speed backfired on us.

Because vaccines traditionally took five to ten years to be approved for use in humans, we had never before gotten a vaccine ready in time to be used while the pandemic was active. Doing so this time opened a Pandora's Box. Had Mrs. Wojcicki and others at YouTube not prohibited the world from gaining the knowledge that vaccination was not necessary to reach herd immunity, the problems we're having now, including the deaths, would be far fewer in number, perhaps non-existent.

Finally, I used this pair of diagrams to show that the vaccine did not prevent people from getting or spreading the virus. I did this in mid-January, 2021. Unfortunately for the people misled into getting the vaccine , Drs. Fauci and Walensky continued with their false information for six more months, claiming, "if you get vaccinated, you cannot get infected or spread the virus to another person.; you are a 'dead end'". Lots of Cable and network TV hosts did the same. Rachel Maddow stood out among this group because of her considerable communication skills but all of them did it. I believe they were just parroting Drs. Fauci and Walensky since they couldn't have figured it out on their own. Clearly, Drs. Fauci and Walensky couldn't either, unless they were lying on purpose, knowing this information would likely have brought vaccine uptake to an abrupt halt. Why would anyone get a vaccine that didn't prevent the recipient from getting infected and therefore could not contribute to herd immunity (which we had already reached, anyway), moreover, an experimental vaccine, never before approved for use in humans and about which, side effects were completely unknown?

I had seen the truth in the data; that the rate of reduction in spread was not great enough. I did so by analyzing data from Israel, as they were ahead of us in getting vaccines into peoples' arms. Before the end of January, the signal was apparent from US data as well. But nobody picked up on it. It wasn't easy to see. You had to look for the rate of reduction in spread taking into account the percent of people who had immunity-in-place, realizing that when a person with immunity-in-place got vaccinated, he wouldn't be spreading the virus to someone else, not because of being vaccinated but because of his immunity-in-place. Since so many experts and everyday clinicians had overlooked immunity-in-place, they weren't able to figure this out. I wish people had seen my video. Most would have decided against the vaccine and many lives would have been saved. The medical community at large finally did pick up on it in April, as the data started to become more clear. Nevertheless, Drs. Fauci and Walensky continued until at least July. Please note the date of the video below. January 24, 2021

▶ YouTube   dr reid sheftall truth in science   ✕   C

4. If we can get infected and spread the virus AFTER we've been vaccinated, why are the airlines saying we have to show a negative test OR be vaccinated before we can get on a plane?

ANS) Yes, isn't that absurdly illogical? They want to put unexposed people on the plane with people who can spread the virus to them and make them deathly ill. It would make much more sense to allow on the planes, only those people who were exposed and recovered from the virus (or never got symptoms). Those people have not gotten infected again, save for 24 out of 800 million worldwide.

MUST WATCH! Vaccine Update! 1.25.2021 Do the Vaccines work?

1,232 views · Jan 24, 2021   👍 73   👎 DISLIKE   ⇗ SHARE   ⬇ DOWNLOAD   ✂ CLIP   ≡+ SAVE   ...

   Dr. Reid Sheftall Truth in Science

3.

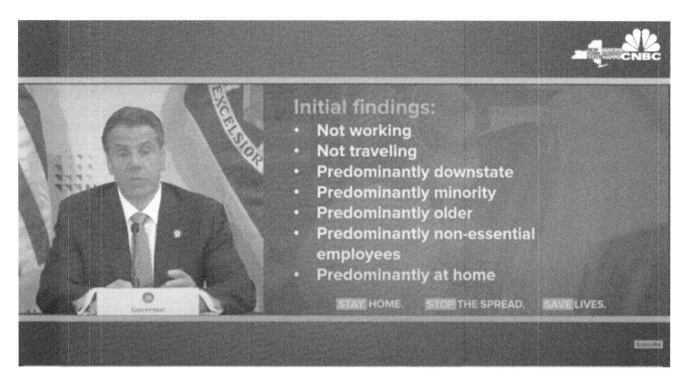

I actually saw this live from Asia. Governor Cuomo was trying to explain two completely contradictory things on the same slide. The findings listed there were characteristics of the people who were faring worse- going to the hospital more often and dying more often. "Predominantly older", "predominantly minority", sure, it makes sense.

Wait! "Predominantly at home"??"Predominantly AT HOME??"People at home were supposed to be doing better! That was the whole point of the lockdowns, right? That may have been the *reason* for locking everyone inside their houses, but was not at all the result they got. They actually got the *opposite* of what they thought would result. Their line of reasoning was faulty. Bringing 18 year-olds home from college where they had contracted COVID and forcing them to lock down with grandma in the stagnant air pocket we call home was just about the stupidest thing you could possibly have done. But that's exactly what lockdown policy effectuated.

The reason this obscure little slide is ranked so high in importance is because it should have alerted the authorities that lockdowns were not working and they should have discontinued the lockdowns from that point forward. But, as far as I can tell, I'm the only person who noticed this. Isn't the tag line "Stay Home. Save Lives" a nice touch, only one centimeter below the data showing people who were predominantly at home died more often?

The point of the lockdowns might have been to protect the public, but that is not what happened. The truth is, they were causing more hospitalization and death, and I'm *not* talking about collateral damage which was enormous. I'm saying the lockdowns caused more hospitalization and death *in and of themselves*. Supporters of the Narrative went ballistic when the results of the study by the Johns Hopkins professor was released. It showed a tiny .2% benefit of lockdowns. Wait until they see this slide.

You have to wonder why Cuomo got involved in trying to explain something that he did not understand at all, something that his medical advisors didn't understand either. To this day, not a single other person in the world understands it. It's one of my "Onlys". We'll get to the explanation shortly. But first, let's say a thing or two about the perils that befall politicians when they try to play doctor.

Remember Governor Cuomo sitting on stage every night giving those COVID-19 briefings that everyone thought were so great? He received an International Emmy Award for his "Masterful COVID-19 briefings" and "in recognition of his leadership during the COVID-19 pandemic and his masterful use of television to inform and calm people around the world." Vanity Fair ran a feature story! NPR talked him up on their morning show! He was lauded in the New York Times and Washington Post! On CNN, there was Avenati-esque talk of him being a shoe-in for the next Democratic Presidential nomination. There was even some behind the scenes talk of him replacing Joe Biden on the 2020 Democratic ticket when Biden's mental deterioration limited his ability to campaign.

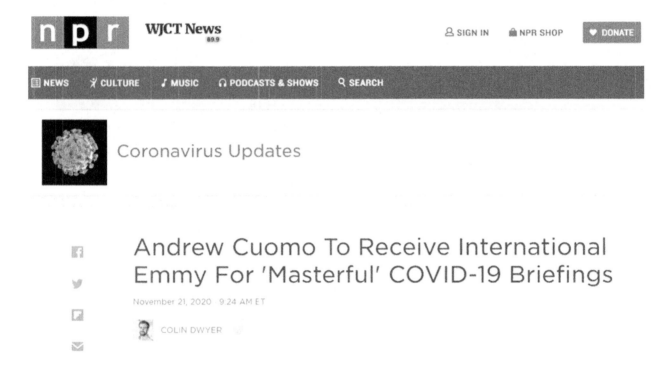

Andrew Cuomo To Receive International Emmy For 'Masterful' COVID-19 Briefings

November 21, 2020 9:24 AM ET

COLIN DWYER

"Thank you to all the members of the Academy. Your work has brought smiles and hope and relief for so many people during these difficult days," Cuomo said. "I wish I could say that my daily COVID presentations are well-choreographed, scripted, rehearsed, or reflected any of the talents you advance. They didn't. They offered only one thing: authentic truth and stability. But sometimes that's enough."

"Authentic truth"? Unfortunately, they offered nothing of the kind. Virtually everything he said was incorrect and the actions he took that arose out of those briefings ended up being very destructive.

I remember standing in front of my TV in Phnom Penh, Cambodia, watching those live briefings every morning before going to the hospital and thinking to myself, "He's got it all wrong. This is not going to end well. I felt bad for him. He had to be getting cleared to say those idiotic things by his medical advisors, at least at first. Later, when he thought he understood some of it, he ventured off into things like why lockdowns would "flatten the curve". Lockdowns were not capable of flattening the curve but both he and his medical advisors didn't understand why. Lockdowns, in fact make things slightly worse as the graphic of Cuomo on CNBC clearly shows. I shouldn't have been so hard on Governor Cuomo because no one else understood why lockdowns could never work, that there never was and there wasn't ever going to be, any "flattening of the curve".

Most will recall that there was an urgency to acquire ventilators in the early days. Cuomo was at the forefront of that effort. Patients with low O2, but who had no difficulty breathing, did not need ventilators; 80% so-treated, died. But the government agreed to pay $38,000 of taxpayer money to the treating hospital for every patient put on a ventilator, and this was after President Trump had given them enormous rescue packages, also using taxpayer money. The patients with low O2 but no difficulty breathing needed high-flow nasal cannulas. 95% of similar patients treated this way, survived. Speaking of ventilators, Governor Cuomo spent $69 million up front to some guy who told his staff on twitter he could fill the order at something like three times the price of a top-of-the-line one and Cuomo agreed. The guy who was a bit of a Silicon Valley hustler hadn't ever put together a ventilator it turns out and still hadn't by the end of the few critical months when there was a short supply. Sixty-nine million to play phone tag for a few months. Not bad work if you can get it. No big deal. It wasn't *his* money and, oh yeah, there was no shortage of ICU beds in NYC hospitals necessitating shipment of COVID-infected patients back to nursing homes. I'm sure you'll recall the Hope Ships waiting in New York Harbor for the overflow that never came (so they turned around after a few weeks and went home).

VANITY FAIR

Andrew Cuomo Accepts Emmy Award as Coronavirus Cases Continue to Rise

The Governor of New York was honored for the viral press conferences he held in the early stages of the pandemic, and was feted by a host of New York stars, including Spike Lee, Ben Stiller, and Robert De Niro.

BY CHRISTOPHER ROSEN
NOVEMBER 24, 2020

I wonder if Spike Lee, Ben Stiller, and Robert De Niro knew those briefings by Governor Cuomo were composed of nonsense. Every time I heard those briefings, I said to myself, "A politician playing doctor... What could go wrong?"

Start with the nursing home deaths, estimated to be 25,000 people including the contributions from three governors (Whitmer of Michigan, Murphy of New Jersey, and Wolf of Pennsylvania) who took Cuomo's lead. That's almost 150 times as many as were killed by Timothy McVeigh in Oklahoma City on April 19, 1995. It's more than the top 1,000 serial killers in U.S. history... combined.

4.

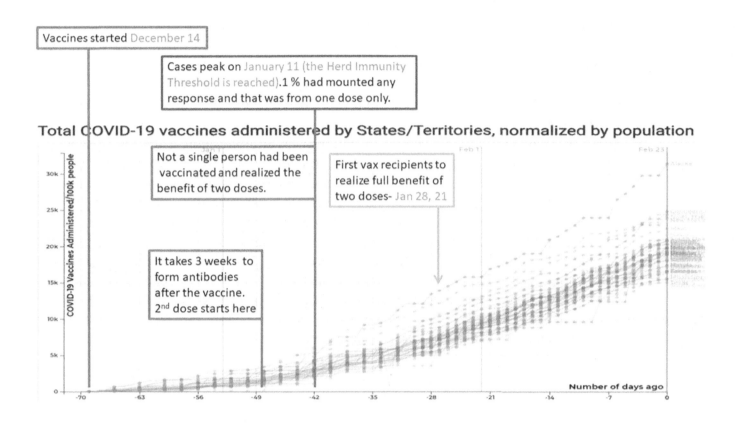

Vaccines started December 14

Cases peak on January 11 (the Herd Immunity Threshold is reached).1 % had mounted any response and that was from one dose only.

Total COVID-19 vaccines administered by States/Territories, normalized by population

Not a single person had been vaccinated and realized the benefit of two doses.

First vax recipients to realize full benefit of two doses- Jan 28, 21

It takes 3 weeks to form antibodies after the vaccine. 2nd dose starts here

Number of days ago

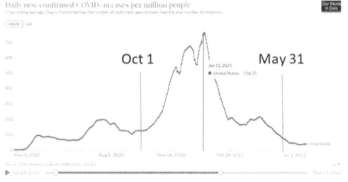

Daily new confirmed COVID-19 cases per million people

Oct 1   May 31

Is January 11 near the end of Flu season?

In the United States, the flu season is considered October through May. It typically reaches an apex in February

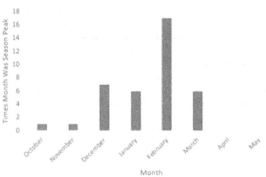

- Was the seasonal bump over? No.
- Did it get unseasonally warm and sunny? No.
- Did they change the cycle threshold on the PCR test? Not until later.
- Did mask wearing, lockdowns, and social distancing finally have an effect? Don't be stupid.
- Oh , it was the Vaccines! No, the Vaccines Had NOTHING TO DO WITH THE DROPS IN CASES, HOSPITALIZATIONS, AND DEATHS!

As far as I know, no one else has recognized or acknowledged that we reached herd immunity on January 11, 2021 for the Wuhan strain.

Could I be wrong such that there is another reason why the case dropped off in the middle of the season? One possibility is that the winter season ended. That's not it. The winter season doesn't end until the end of May. Was it a very warm winter that "tricked" the virus into thinking the season had ended? No, this was the year Texas got so cold in February their electric grid almost failed! Remember Ted Cruz getting in trouble because his wife flew to Cancun to get out of the cold? Could changing the threshold of the PCR test have done it?- Yes, but this wasn't done until later. Could it have dropped because masks, lockdowns, and social distancing finally had an effect on the curve? Don't be stupid. What about the vaccines? We started administering them on December 14, 2020. No, only 1% of the population had gotten a single shot. Not even one person had gotten the benefit of being fully-vaccinated; NOT ONE PERSON!

The graph dropped off like that because we reached herd immunity. Not a single person in the world recognized this at the time or has recognized it now, (another of my "Onlys"). We still hear "experts" talking about us "never being able to reach herd immunity" when the truth is, we've reached it for the Wuhan, Alpha, Delta, and Omicron strains; and all without a single person contributing to the herd because of vaccination. (please see the next slide.)

How did we reach herd immunity on January 11, 2021? Here are the numbers as of September 28, 2020. At least 40% of the U.S. population had immunity-in-place according to the second most important slide of the pandemic. (According to the slide it is more like 50%, but we'll stay conservative) The U.S. population including undocumented people is 365 million. 40% of that is 146 million. About 155 million people had been exposed to the virus by then, not the 9 million confirmed exposures Johns Hopkins put on the CNN ticker that day. I know this because the WHO informed us that 10% of the world population had been exposed on that day. Since the world population was about 7.85 billion at that time, 785 million had been exposed worldwide. But Hopkins claimed 45.7 million had been exposed worldwide. So they were undercounting exposures by a factor of 17.2. (In fairness to Hopkins, they counted only *confirmed* exposures. That's partially responsible for why they were always so far off). To arrive at the correct number of exposed in the U.S., we need only multiply Hopkins's number of 9 million by the Hopkins undercounting factor of 17.2 to get the actual number. This product is 155 million. Our total number in the herd on September 28, 2020 was 146 million + 155 million = 301 million. We got the other 50 million or so necessary for us to reach the herd immunity threshold during that first winter season, from September 28, 2020 to January 11, 2021 and the cases vs. time came tumbling down, never to be seen again.

It's worth noting that Dr. Fauci and the rest of the M.D.T.V. mafia were claiming only 9% had been exposed and 91% were vulnerable in late September of 2020. They were basing their claims on serology tests- checking the blood for the presence of antibodies- not realizing that people can be protected having recovered from the disease even if they have very low or no antibodies in their blood. Antibodies only last for about 90 days in the blood. People who got sick and recovered more than 90 days previous to their sampling, would be missed. Those people who have recovered from the disease have clonal memory and are protected from getting infected and spreading it to someone else. They are, therefore, part of the herd. Second, they are neglecting T-cell protection by only checking for antibodies in the blood. And last, but certainly not least, they were not counting patients with immunity-in-place when they claimed 91% of the population was still vulnerable and we were very far from herd immunity. We were actually very close to herd immunity, and reached it in the middle of the upcoming winter season as I have shown.

From the beginning of the pandemic, the experts ignored T cells. This was a major oversight. For viral infections, T-Cells are more important than B-cells. B-cells need T-helper cells to be activated fully. T-cells, on the other hand, do not need B-cells. They can operate at maximum efficiency on their own.

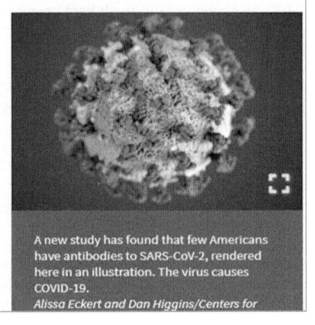
Here is an article about the Parsonnet study that drew so many incorrect conclusions such as "about 9% of the people have been infected with the coronavirus" and "we are nowhere near herd immunity". This happened because they only considered people who had antibodies in their blood as being part of the herd.

5.

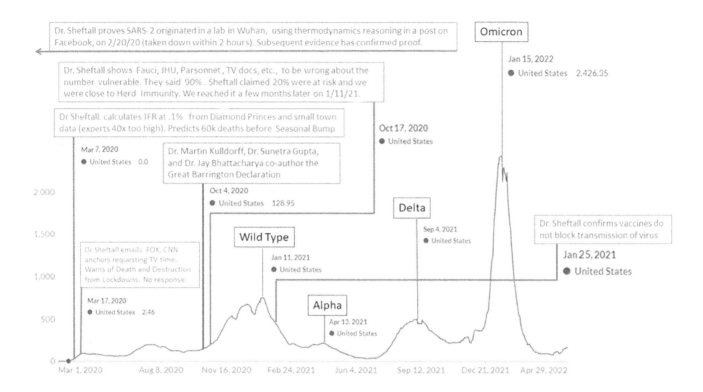

This graph and the slide below (which offers the detailed explanation) show that we reached herd immunity for each of the wild type, alpha, delta and omicron variants without the help of vaccinations. (Since vaccines don't block transmission, they couldn't possibly contribute to herd immunity.) The dates at which we reached herd immunity are in the graph and description below. (Note: I made this slide for Dr. Jay Bhattacharya as a "thank you" for our 24 hours of video discussions together, thus, the flags marking our major discoveries.)

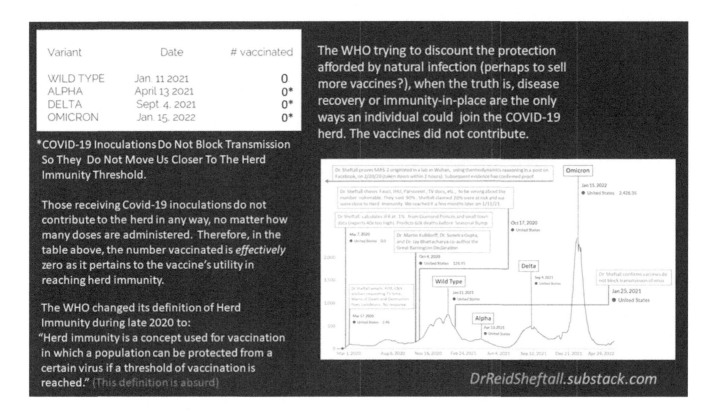

Variant	Date	# vaccinated
WILD TYPE	Jan. 11 2021	0
ALPHA	April 13 2021	0*
DELTA	Sept. 4, 2021	0*
OMICRON	Jan. 15, 2022	0*

The WHO trying to discount the protection afforded by natural infection (perhaps to sell more vaccines?), when the truth is, disease recovery or immunity-in-place are the only ways an individual could join the COVID-19 herd. The vaccines did not contribute.

*COVID-19 Inoculations Do Not Block Transmission So They Do Not Move Us Closer To The Herd Immunity Threshold.

Those receiving Covid-19 inoculations do not contribute to the herd in any way, no matter how many doses are administered. Therefore, in the table above, the number vaccinated is *effectively* zero as it pertains to the vaccine's utility in reaching herd immunity.

The WHO changed its definition of Herd Immunity during late 2020 to:
"Herd immunity is a concept used for vaccination in which a population can be protected from a certain virus if a threshold of vaccination is reached." (This definition is absurd)

DrReidSheftall.substack.com

This is incredibly important because it shows we never needed a single person vaccinated to reach herd immunity for any of the variants we have encountered. All of the talk from Dr. Fauci, Dr. Birx, Bill Gates, Joe Biden, Dr. Peter Hotez, the rest of the M.D.T.V. Mafia that we needed 60 – 70%, and then 90% and finally 98% of the population vaccinated to reach herd immunity was utter nonsense.

6.

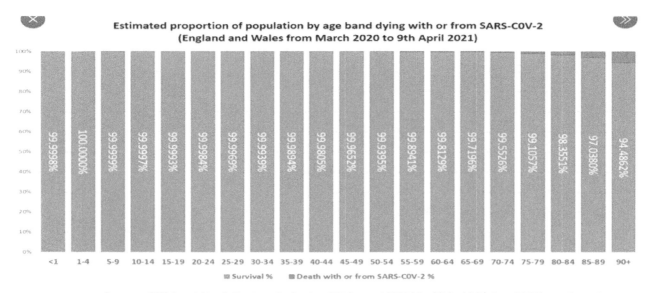

Estimated proportion of population by age band dying with or from SARS-COV-2
(England and Wales from March 2020 to 9th April 2021)

Age band	Survival %
<1	99.9998%
1-4	100.0000%
5-9	99.9999%
10-14	99.9997%
15-19	99.9993%
20-24	99.9984%
25-29	99.9969%
30-34	99.9939%
35-39	99.9894%
40-44	99.9805%
45-49	99.9652%
50-54	99.9395%
55-59	99.8941%
60-64	99.8129%
65-69	99.7196%
70-74	99.5526%
75-79	99.1057%
80-84	98.3551%
85-89	97.0380%
90+	94.4862%

■ Survival %　■ Death with or from SARS-COV-2 %

Sources: ONS Population Estimates... England and Wales....mid 2019 (published 24th June 2020): unadjusted
ONS Deaths Registered Weekly to 9th April 2021 - covid19 occurrence data (published 20th April 2021)

England and Wales ONS Data. This Bar graph tells us that if you were under 80 years of age, your chances of dying of COVID-19 is less than one in a hundred and that's "with" or "from" SARS-2. Our politicians and some evil business people with the help of the lettered agencies (CDC, FDA, NIH) and the MSM shut down the world, causing death and destruction on a massive scale, for almost no slivers of red in the under 65 working age group.

7.

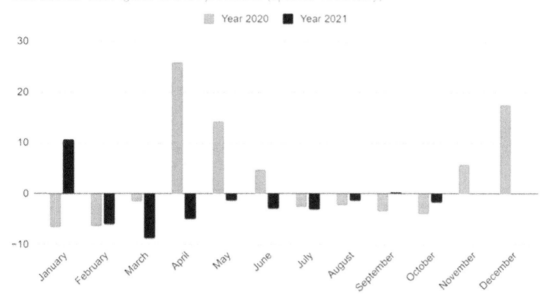

Deviation from average death per month of 2015-2019 per 100 000

Data Source: SCB, figures for 2021 provisional (updated 10 January)

Year 2020   Year 2021

        The first thing that struck me about this graph was that, in both 2020 and 2021, more than half the months had deaths per 100,000 *lower* than the average of 2015 to 2019.
In a PANDEMIC? You've got to be kidding me! Then I looked at the worst month, April of 2020. The graph shows that SWEDEN, in that month, only experienced 26 excess deaths per one hundred thousand people.
26/100,000 = .00026 = .026 %
In other words, at the worst time of the pandemic, the deaths per 100,000 people went up only 2.6 hundredths of 1 %.
That's what we stopped the world for.

Let's gather some more amazing information, this time using the entire graph.
        Back to the first shocking fact… During the entire two years shown, in only six of the 24 months was the bar in positive territory while in 15 months there were actually fewer deaths than the average of 2015 – 2019, and in three there were essentially the same. And remember, this was when the much more virulent Wuhan strain predominated. Carefully adding up the totals for the six bars above the line and subtracting the 15 bars below the line gives us 40 deaths total. Remember, we're counting per 100,000 population. Still, there are 24 months. 40/24 = 1.67. In a country that eschewed lockdowns, masks, social distancing and school closures, an additional 1.67 out of 100,000 people died per month.

That's .0000167 or .00167%. This is for Sweden, remember, the "control group" for the world. It means, per month, for the two worst years of the pandemic (2020 and 2021) and fighting the most virulent variant, the original Wuhan strain, only 1/6th of 1% of 1% per 100,000 people died in excess of the average from 2015 – 2019 (before the pandemic existed). For Sweden… the country that eschewed lockdowns, mask mandates, and school closures, where women walked arm-in-arm down the street past bars full of screaming fans, beers in hand, to enjoy a dinner and a movie together in a crowded theater.

That's right. I saw videos of all this on CNN. 1/6th of 1% of 1% per 100,000 people more in a given month than died BEFORE THE PANDEMIC STARTED! And it would have been a lot less if Sweden had not had such a mild flu season the previous winter, leaving many more than the average number of the very elderly and vulnerable to face COVID-19 when it did finally come.

Again, this is what Birx, Fauci and others shut down the entire world for AND for which they destroyed lives and forced a toxic vaccine into the arms of people (including children) who didn't understand this stuff and relied on them for guidance. With people like Peter Hotez saying the way Trump was managing the pandemic was a threat to our Homeland security. Really, Dr. Hotez? .0000167 per 100,000 people per month? The people who did this should be put in prison for life and everyone who profited from this crime should be forced to return the money a la the Bernie Madoff scandal beneficiaries.

… and I hate to add insult to injury for those who think this was a "once-in-a-century disaster" such as Bill Gates and many others including CNN and MSNBC Hosts, but all of this includes "with" as well as "from" COVID. In other words, a lot of those 1/6th of 1% of 1% people died of something other than COVID-19 but were recorded that way because they had a positive PCR test which, very likely, was a false positive. (Please see *5 Reasons Why Calling a Positive PCR Result a "New Case", Should Be Punishable By Death"*)

Sweden's population is 10.35 million which equals 103.5 x 100,000. So there are 103.5 "units of 100,000" there. The number of such units in the official U.S. population is 3,300. Taking Sweden's number of 40 deaths/100,000 over the two years x 3,300 gives a total death count "with" and "from" COVID of 132,000 for the U.S. During the same time, 840,000 deaths were assigned to COVID in the U.S.

There are a few reasons why our death count should be higher than Sweden's. We are fatter and sicker in the U.S. That might account for 20 or 30 percent more in the U.S but the U.S. total is about 6.5 times that of Sweden. What is going on? Why is there such a huge discrepancy?

The lion's share of the difference is because we exaggerated our deaths in the U.S. Our government gave perverse monetary incentives to call a death a "COVID death" when a 40 cycle PCR was positive as Dr. Ezike pointed out so bravely, "Even when there was a clear alternative cause of death, if they tested positive for COVID, it was recorded as a COVID death". (Please see slide #1 in this section, where I show the guidelines for assigning the cause of death was changed on March 24, 2020 from what was used the previous 17 years such that by August 28, we had assigned 16.7 times as many deaths to COVID-19 than we would have if the guidelines hadn't been changed.)

Sweden had a disproportionate number of deaths in their nursing homes, largely because they had a very mild flu season the year before and there were many vulnerable people still alive who would have normally succumbed a year earlier. Those patients were very old and fragile and had several co-morbidities. It is very hard to tell if a patient like this is dying of COVID or one of their co-morbidities. Sweden probably exaggerated their deaths also but to not nearly the same extent as the U.S.

8.

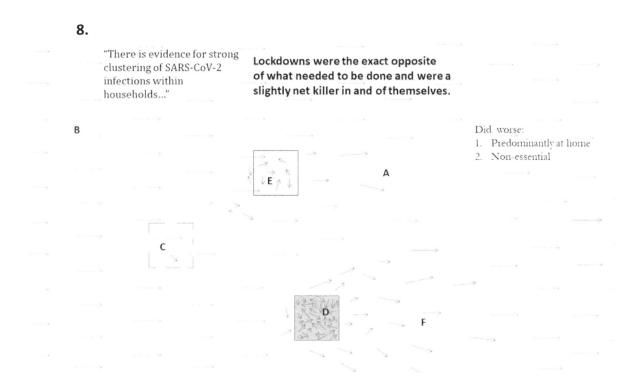

"There is evidence for strong clustering of SARS-CoV-2 infections within households..."

Lockdowns were the exact opposite of what needed to be done and were a slightly net killer in and of themselves.

B

Did worse:
1. Predominantly at home
2. Non-essential

A

E

C

D

F

Dr. Robert Redfield, our former CDC Director, said in Senate testimony while holding up a surgical mask, "Masks are the most important, powerful, public health tool we have." The degree of stupidity and laziness associated with this disaster of management that was COVID-19, is almost inconceivable. If Dr. Redfield couldn't figure this out on his own, he could have watched one of my videos or looked at the literature which showed meta-analyses covering randomized, controlled trials over 72 years, all of which showed no significant reduction in transmission of laboratory-confirmed influenza.

The best thing you could do during the pandemic was get outside in the sunshine, exercise and lose some weight. If the sunshine wasn't enough to get your vitamin D level up to around 50 ng/ml, you needed to take a supplement.

COVID-19 is a disease of the vascular endothelium. It is not a pulmonary disease as was first suspected. I'll leave the technical reasoning behind this conclusion for my next book. For now, suffice it to say, with diseases like this, the best things you can do are exercise and lose weight, get your blood sugar in order and lower your blood pressure if it is elevated. I believe that the increased mortality from COVID in black males can be accounted for, primarily, by the tendency toward higher blood pressure in that group. How many black men in their 50s die suddenly because of complications from unchecked hypertension? It's a disgrace. We need to STOP using the health of black men to push some kind of political agenda in saying that the main reason black men had higher rates of death from COVID is because black people are discriminated against in our healthcare system. That exists but it is a very minor factor. Start recognizing the real reason; the fact that many black men have dangerously-high blood pressure, exacerbating the damage the spike proteins do to the vascular endothelium. These men need treatment, not all talk and no action by social justice warriors on the internet. The virtue signalers are pushing a real health problem to the back burner when they try to attribute everything to social issues. I have no doubt that their concerns are genuine, but they are hurting the black community in the process by turning the emphasis away from a real problem that is devastating that community.

In yet another bonehead move a la Dr. Redfield's total lack of understanding of mask science, the government put lockdowns in place. I blame Dr. Birx, primarily, but Anthony Fauci, Matthew Pottinger, and others for the death and destruction caused by this horrendous decision by Trump.

The COVID-19 response team recommend locking down, and Trump went along with it- the exact *opposite* of what needed to be done, by locking us in our homes. To make sure no one went outside to exercise, they padlocked the entrances to public parks. Just in case someone got in anyway, they nailed boards over basketball hoops at God knows what expense to the public.

The diagram above explains why lockdowns are the opposite of what should be done in a pandemic caused by a respiratory virus. **C** is a well-ventilated house with windows open everywhere. The owners understand the principle that you want to keep the concentration of virus particles as low as possible by making the indoors as much like the outdoors as possible. There was evidence that this was the correct line of reasoning from the beginning, such as, 1) data that showed the people doing the worst were people <u>predominantly at home</u> and people who were <u>non-essential employees,</u> (but nobody except for me seemed to notice this and when I called attention to it, YouTube took my videos down or shadow banned me) and 2) the realization that most infections were occurring in the home (where the stagnant air was, OF COURSE).

When windows are closed in a house, stagnant air is created inside. Virus accumulates in stagnant air in the same way that runners will spend more time in a soft, sandy portion of a long distance race, per unit distance, than they do running on a hard surface.

Pretend you are staging a marathon by having runners go 105 times around a 400 meter track where a 100 meter section has been removed and replaced with soft, 10 inch deep, dry beach sand, the kind you sink 4 inches into every time you take a step. If you take a snapshot of the entire course, say 30 laps into the race, you would see more runners in the soft sandy portion than in any other 100 meter section of the track.

When you have a virus that is transmitted by aerosols, particles stay in the air for hours or days. The best way to get them out is to increase the ventilation. Stagnant air is your enemy. Virus particles will accumulate there.

The stagnant air scenario is depicted by **E**, a poorly-ventilated house with a concentration three or four times higher than that of the outside. **D** depicts a house where one of the inhabitants is infected with the virus. It is not ventilated properly and is filling with virus. That is a particularly dangerous house to be living in. Even opening the side windows would help enormously in such a house if the wind is blowing outside as air would get sucked out in accordance with Bernoulli's principle, in the same way that cracking a window relieves a closed, fast moving car of smoke inside. It is the same principle that causes the plastic curtain to keep coming in and hitting you when you are taking a shower.

9.

The conclusions that can be drawn from slide 7 should convince you that the pandemic wasn't exactly a "nothing-burger" but it was pretty close. Given the shocking numbers that led to those conclusions and that there were no recorded flu deaths that year, COVID-19 probably would have come and gone without people noticing if the government and special interests hadn't inflated the deaths by changing the guidelines for assigning cause of death, if they hadn't used the PCR test to find so-called "new cases" and if they hadn't imposed all of the destructive policies on everyone. Lots of deceit and criminal activity occurred.

If I hadn't witnessed it, I never would have believed that people who are reasonably intelligent and function pretty well in their day-to-day lives could have fallen for this. There are still huge numbers of the population, University administrators and students, medical doctors, including heads of virology departments at major hospitals who think it was all legit. These people believe the Chinese videos of people keeling over in the streets from COVID are real. They believe Bill Gates was lucky when he picked an obscure German biotech company named BioNTech from a pool of 1,000 similar companies back in September of 2019. This was before their stock traded publically and three months before China would announce to the world in late December that they had discovered their first case of viral pneumonia caused by a new coronavirus. China said the new coronavirus did not transmit from person to person.; Gates said that he had no advanced knowledge that a virus had escaped (or was released) and already circulating through the population and that BioNTech was going to partner with Pfizer to distribute vaccines for that virus all over the world for the foreseeable future. They believe the inserts into the SARS-2 genome got there by some process with which we are not yet familiar. Perhaps most telling, they believe the U.S. had 6.5 times as many cases of COVID-19 per capita compared to a country that did not use lockdowns while at the same time, believing lockdowns work.

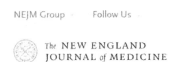
Perspective

Responding to Covid-19 — A Once-in-a-Century Pandemic?

Bill Gates

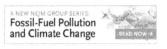

IN ANY CRISIS, LEADERS HAVE TWO EQUALLY IMPORTANT RESPONSIBILITIES: SOLVE the immediate problem and keep it from happening again. The Covid-19 pandemic is a case in point. We need to save lives now while also improving the way we respond to outbreaks in general. The first point is more pressing, but the second has crucial long-term consequences.

The long-term challenge — improving our ability to respond to outbreaks — isn't new. Global health experts have been saying for years that another pandemic whose speed and severity rivaled those of the committed substantial resources in recent years to helping the world prepare for such a scenario.

Now we also face an immediate crisis. In the past week, Covid-19 has started behaving a lot like the once-in-a-century pathogen we've been worried about. I hope it's not that bad, but we should assume it will be until we know otherwise.

There are two reasons that Covid-19 is such a threat. First, it can kill healthy adults in addition to elderly people with existing health problems. The data so far suggest that the virus has a case fatality risk around 1%; this rate would make it many times more severe than typical seasonal influenza, putting it somewhere between the 1957 influenza pandemic (0.6%) and the 1918 influenza pandemic (2%).[2]

Second, Covid-19 is transmitted quite efficiently. The average infected person spreads the disease to two

Billions of dollars for antipandemic efforts is a lot of money. But that's the scale of investment required to solve the problem. And given the economic pain that an epidemic can impose — we're already seeing how Covid-19 can disrupt supply chains and stock markets, not to mention people's lives — it will be a bargain.

Finally, governments and industry will need to come to an agreement: during a pandemic, vaccines and antivirals can't simply be sold to the highest bidder. They should be available and affordable for people who are at the heart of the outbreak and in greatest need. Not only is such distribution the right thing to do, it's also the right strategy for short-circuiting transmission and preventing future pandemics.

These are the actions that leaders should be taking now. There is no time to waste.

The New England Journal of Medicine used to be one of the two most prestigious medical journals in the world. Everyone knows Bill. He is a brilliant man with an exceptional track record in business but is this the place for him to be sharing his ideas? These few paragraphs display a lack of medical perspective commonly seen in non-medical people. He tells us "we face an immediate crisis." No, no. The next sentence, is even worse. "In the past week, COVID-19 has started behaving a lot like the once-in-a-century pathogen we've been worried about." No, no

I'd like to know the evidence upon which he based these extreme assertions. I'm not going to get it from Gates. He should have shared the evidence and reasoning that gave rise to this article but he didn't so I'll look for the case and death numbers for February 20 – 27 as this article was published on February 28. OK, I went to Our World in Data. There weren't any cases or deaths between February 20 and February 27, 2020. So we know he didn't base the "Pandemic of the Century on cases and deaths."

Reading further down, (with my reaction in bold) he writes, "There are two reasons (why) COVID-19 is such a threat. First, it can kill healthy adults in addition to elderly people with existing health problems. [**This is a meaningless statement. It is true of the seasonal flu and the common cold too.**] Then Bill talks about the case fatality rate. He makes the point that a CFR of 1% (which is fairly close to the actual number) is many times more severe than a typical seasonal influenza. I'll have to address this two ways because I don't know if Bill is getting the CFR confused with the IFR or not. First assuming he means as he says, that the CFR for SARS-2 is many times higher than the CFR for seasonal influenza. He's right but it doesn't mean SARS-2 is any worse. In this case, it means there are a lot more asymptomatic cases in SARS-2 than the flu (where there are almost none.) Remember, for something to be a case, symptoms must be present. With SARS-2, there are many, many asymptomatic infections. The IFR and CFR for the flu are the same because you always get symptoms with the Flu. The infection fatality rate IFR of the flu is .1% as it is for SARS-2. CFR = IFR for the flu because everyone gets symptoms with the flu. For SARS-2, the IFR is .1% but the CFR is about 1%. Now I'll answer under the assumption that Bill is getting his terms mixed up. If Bill was writing "CFR" but meant "IFR", he's in error. The IFR for SARS-2 was .1% for all age groups (higher for the elderly, particularly, those over 80 years old where it can get up to around 10%) and 1,000 to about 10,000 times lower in small children where the risk is down to about 1 in a million. There's nothing meaningful there either. The rest of the the article talks about how much money it's going to take and that it's a good investment.

OK, there were no cases and no deaths during the week he is referring to. SARS-2 has a miniscule IFR in healthy adult males. So that meant nothing. It looks like there was no useful information and he didn't support his claims at all that SARS-2 might causative agent in a once-in-a-century pandemic. So after he makes an effort to scare people, he talks about the government needing to spend a lot of money on this and tells people it will be a good investment.

You have to blame the NEJM for printing an article like this. It was devoid of anything useful and was incorrect in a few places. Gates may not know this. He might have thought it was helpful.

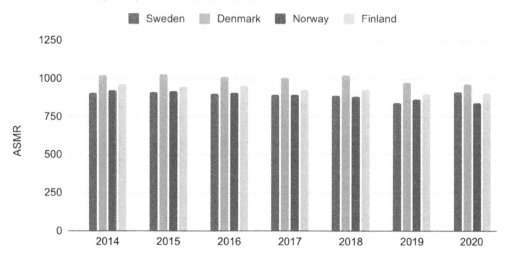

A Once in a Century Pandemic??

The four Scandinavian countries had fewer deaths in 2020, the worst year of the pandemic, than in any other year since 2014. If you don't think you were taken for a ride over this, you have lost your ability to interpret data that doesn't agree with your political ideology or some other built-in bias. This fraud, and "fraud" is the correct word because reality was misrepresented by your own government, the M.D.T.V. Mafia, the MSM, and medical doctors, epidemiologists, and public health workers everywhere who supported the Narrative.

10 Reasons Why We Could Eradicate Small Pox But Not COVID-19

1. **The Small Pox virus does not exist in any animal reservoir; only in humans.** Dogs, cats, lions, tigers... Lots of animals now harbor SARS-2. Something like 80% of the white-tailed deer population carry it.

2. **It was easy to see who was infected with the small pox viruses, variola major and minor, because every infected person exhibited an obvious pock mark rash characterized by oozing pustules.** You can't tell who is infected with Sars-2 or who has recovered from COVID-19 just by looking.

3. **No laboratory tests were required to confirm infection with variola. Presence of the typical rash confirmed the diagnosis.** You need a lab test to confirm COVID-19 notwithstanding all the hospital physicians and billing departments who just wrote it down.

4. **A freeze-dried vaccine was developed which could withstand temperatures up to 98 degrees Fahrenheit for a month. It did not have to be stored at 70 degrees below zero like mRNA vaccines.** Lots of money has been wasted due to careless handling of the vaccines. They had to be discarded because the very low temperature was not maintained.

5. **The small pox vaccine was the live-attenuated type.** The COVID-19 vaccines used in the US, Canada, Europe and South America were mRNA vaccines (Pfizer, Moderna) or viral vector vaccines (Astra-Zeneca, Johnson and Johnson).

6. **Successfully-vaccinated people could not spread the disease to others.** Not so for the COVID-19 vaccines

7. **The vaccine was very inexpensive.** Ha-ha Wait until the medical bills come in for sick vaccine recipients.

8. **A single shot conferred immunity for at least 10 years.** Ha-ha

9. **Every successful vaccination developed into a pustule at the injection site and then a distinctive scar, making it easy to see who had been vaccinated.** You can't tell who was vaccinated for COVID-19 by looking. It wouldn't do you any good if you could.

10. **Teams surveying an area could easily tell whether Small pox had been there, when it was there, who was vaccinated and who had recovered from the disease.** Not so for COVID-19.

3 Types of Viral Gain of Function Research (VGOF) Considered Acceptable by the International Community

1. Receptor Binding Domain Optimization (changing the animal it can infect)

2. Increasing the infectivity of the virus

3. Increasing the pathogenicity of the virus

2 That are Not

These are not allowed because their only application is in the creation of bio-weapons.

1. Gain of Function that makes Asymptomatic Transmission possible.

In my opinion, this is the most interesting kind of gain of function research. It should not have been done with SARS-2, but it was. The result was Open Reading Frame-8 (ORF-8) sitting in the middle of the SARS-2 genome. ORF-8 prevents interferons from mediating pain and sickness. Preventing pain and sickness is good, right? Not in this case. Without the wonderful effects of ORF-8, people get sick and feel uncomfortable, and they look the part. Before antibiotics, and vaccines, getting sick with a contagious infectious disease frequently meant death. So people got very good at avoiding the sick. But you wouldn't know how to avoid people who are asymptomatic. Furthermore, people who are sick and in pain usually go home and stay in bed, away from society. People infected with virus that contains a symptom-buster like ORF-8- aren't at home, sick in bed. They're at a group conference at work in an unventilated room, passing the virus on to everyone there who is vulnerable including secretaries and cleaners who aren't present for the conference but go into the room hours later to tidy up.

You want the sequence of nucleotides in ORF-8 to be in a bio-weapon because it increases the rate of spread. Nobody knows who has it, so vulnerable people don't know who to avoid.

I used to think asymptomatic transmission constituted a first principles violation. The steps a virus takes in going from symbiosis with the reservoir host to being able to be transmitted from human to human must occur in a certain order.

You shouldn't have a virus that can spread from human to human before it causes symptoms. This is because you need more of a viral load to go from human to human than you need to cause symptoms And you actually don't have that. Enter ORF-8, a protein that blocks symptoms. It's a protein that gets synthesized by the virus and sent into the blood before even RNA polymerase gets made. SARS-2 got/gets into a lot of people because even asymptomatic people can spread it. People are asymptomatic because ORF-8 prevents symptom expression, not because they didn't have enough viral load to cause symptoms. There is no first principles violation here. Its very low infection fatality rate of .1%. prevented it from killing more people.

2. Gain of Function that Diminishes the Immune System's Ability to mount a strong response. Again, ORF-8 is the culprit. It inhibits the presentation of peptides on the surface of invaded cells by the Major Histocompatibility Complex (MHC)., Class I for T-killer cells and Class II for T-helper cells. T-helpers won't be able to recognize foreign peptides on the surface of infected cells and stimulate B-cells to differentiate into antibody-producing plasma cells and T-helpers won't be stimulating T-killer cells to recognize the foreign peptide and destroy the invaded cell. You can see why this kind of research is unacceptable. If you can't make antibodies and you can't destroy cells that have been invaded by viruses that hijacked that cell's replication machinery to make copies of themselves, you won't survive an infection with a virulent virus. This is why children who are born without the ability to make T-cells have to live their lives in a plastic bubble because an infection by any routine bacteria or virus will kill them. During discussions with Dr. Steven Quay, I learned about two Masters theses that dealt with making ORF-8 more effective at damaging the human immune system. The papers were not translated into English for obvious reasons but Dr. Quay was able to get them translated. The research associated with the two papers is being conducted at the Wuhan Institute of Virology. This is a very serious violation. These people are not cub scouts and we should *not* be sharing our technology and know-how with them.

7 Idiotic Proposals to Reduce SARS-2 Transmission

1. Lockdowns were the most destructive policy in the history of medicine. The WHO predicted 140 million people will starve to death because of the supply chain disruptions they caused.

The 45 million put to death by Mao Zedong are Girl Scout cookies compared to the number of deaths caused by the lockdown endorsers including Drs. Birx, Fauci, Walensky, Redfield, Wen, Reiner, Hotez, Haseltine, and the rest of the M.D.T.V. Mafia.

OK, so they didn't understand why lockdowns couldn't work early on- I really wouldn't expect them to- but after the data came in, the graphs were unchanged and you couldn't tell which of two neighboring states or countries locked down and which didn't. You must see a jog to a lesser slope when they take effect. We never saw this for any country at any time. Not seeing any benefit graphically, yet seeing enormous cost, should have made Drs. Fauci, Collins, Birx, Walensky, and the rest of the M.D.T.V. Mafia call for the immediate cessation of lockdowns.

See if you can do it. All of these countries used strict lockdowns except one. Which one allowed their citizens to roam about as they pleased? The graphs are of deaths vs. time.

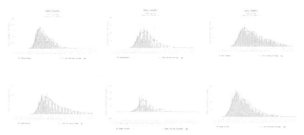

2. Moratoria placed on all but elective surgery. This meant we couldn't biopsy suspicious breast lumps. Those women who lost their jobs and health insurance couldn't afford it anyway, even with surgeons doing the procedures free of charge. I know this from personal experience. I urged women to do this. I offered to do it for them free of charge. Only one or two out of 50 patients took me up on it (because the full work-up involves many other costly things such as mammograms, anesthesia, OR time, pathological examination, etc.)

This boiled over into irrationality regarding other, much more deadly medical conditions. People were terrified of going to the hospital for fear of catching a virus with a one-in-a-thousand infection fatality rate- lower if they were under 65- and neglected conditions that were truly life-threatening. There were even cases of people with severe chest pain refusing to call an ambulance.

Also, people couldn't or wouldn't come in for cancer screening such as colonoscopies and are paying for it now. Many adenocarcinomas that arose from polyps that could have routinely been removed with the scope a few years ago, have now metastasized to the liver, greatly reducing the chance of survival and now involving a major operation. Those who endorsed lockdowns and moratoria on non-emergency surgery are murderers and belong in prison for the rest of their lives.

3. Closing Schools

This wasn't done to reduce transmission or to protect teachers. It was so teachers could get paid while not working. Many teachers got side jobs tutoring groups of children in their homes where the ventilation was worse. It was Randi Weingarten's way of getting her union membership some free money at the taxpayers' expense.

When this was proposed, I made a post explaining if you were going to close the schools for COVID, you would have to close them every year for the flu because flu causes much more morbidity and mortality in this age-group. No one listened. As more and more data came out, showing children were not putting each other or their teachers at increased risk, the abuses continued. Ms. Weingarten lobbied the CDC to keep schools closed. Enormous damage was done to students kept out of school for long periods of time. They will drop out of school more, earn less, are more likely to live in poverty, and will die sooner.

3. Mask use by the general public

Surgical and cloth masks don't block transmission significantly. 72 years of meta-analyses of randomized controlled trials demonstrated this clearly. For some reason, no one took the time to read the literature. They both have enormous holes through which 100 nanometer viruses transmit easily. As with lockdowns, you can't solve a nanoscopic problem with a macroscopic solution! If you're thinking N95 masks would work, forget it. You have to seal N95 masks for them to do very little, if anything. These seals get broken soon after they are made because people cannot tolerate them.

Masks are known to cause problems too. They hinder speech development in some children. They cause acne and tooth decay. They create pockets of stagnant air that trap bacteria and, ironically, some SARS-2 particles, both of which get inhaled back into your lungs on the next breath along with lots of other waste including CO_2.

A surgeon- I can't use his name because I can no longer find this quote- who has appeared repeatedly as a guest expert on many networks promoted mask use by saying, "If it's good enough for surgeons in the O.R., it's good enough for me!" No, doctor. Masks are used as splash guards by surgeons in the O.R., analogous to the reason we wear clear eye protection when sawing bones or operating on patients with AIDS or hepatitis. They also protect patients from doctors who spit when speaking, particularly when they are agitated. Masks make things worse when the surgeon sneezes or coughs because people naturally turn their heads to the side when they do these things. The expelled water droplets containing bacteria and viruses shoot out the sides of the masks through the large openings, right into the patient's open surgical wound.

4. Plexi-glass walls around office workers' desks and in restaurants

These are just little plexi-glass "houses" around your nose and mouth, creating stagnant air for you to breathe for hours every day. These were the opposite of what those workers really needed- small fans to keep the air moving.

5. Closing parks

People should have been outside in the fresh air and sun, increasing their vitamin D levels, breathing low virus concentration, non-stagnant air, getting exercise, losing weight, improving their mental health.

6. Keeping people off of beaches

One of the strangest images I have in my mind is that of a policeman in southern California chasing down the only person on the beach so he could give him a ticket.

7. Plastic curtains placed between grandparents and grandchildren when hugging.

So silly it deserves no comment

9 Most Important Videos of The SARS-2/COVID-19 Era

I'm not including the many outstanding data analysis videos made by well-meaning doctors, data scientists and laymen.

All of these are "must watch".

1. https://www.youtube.com/shorts/ljpHugKNcoI
Dr. Ngozi Ezike's description of how COVID-19 deaths are counted. Everyone in Illinois with a positive test gets COVID-19 recorded as the cause of death even if it could not have made the person die. This occurred everywhere and is commonly referred to as the "with" vs. "from" issue.

2. https://www.youtube.com/watch?v=Y_MeeYbYtWc
Dr. Fauci admitting if you got the disease, you don't need to get the vaccine for influenza. This is the opposite of what he said leading up to vaccine enrollment

3. https://www.youtube.com/watch?v=g5jx243DHyg&t=620s
Mike Wallace's expose of the 1976 Swine Flu fraud. Imagine if we had journalists like this today.

4. https://www.youtube.com/watch?v=Uf4-Vzf1CyM
One of the many fake Chinese videos meant to scare the world into accepting destructive measures such as lockdowns and school closures. Everything China did is consistent with at least some aspect of planning. It all makes sense. First, they claimed an infection fatality rate that, at 4%, was 40 times too high.. Then put videos on the internet that showed people collapsing "from" SARS-2. Then they released videos of citywide pool parties in Wuhan after their lockdowns were over as if to say, "Here's how you solve this horrible problem. Just go into lockdowns! Look how well it worked for us!"

5. https://www.youtube.com/watch?v=KL8SJRBNh_w
Dr. Doshi's turn during Senator Johnson's roundtable on COVID-19.

6. https://www.youtube.com/watch?v=tj6EkqfCRbA
One of many videos of Rachel Maddow's show on MSNBC where she spreads incorrect information that leads to the death of many of her viewers who follow her advice, to, for example, "get the vaccine so you won't be able to spread the virus to someone else." She should have known the vaccines don't prevent the recipient from spreading the virus. I proved it months before using a dull #2 pencil and half a sheet of notebook paper in 10 minutes.

In fairness, none of the wokester show hosts of cable and network TV understand virus transmission well enough to figure out any of this on their own. They're just saying what they're told to say. I don't know what all of their salaries are but it is fairly well-known that Rachel Maddow has 30 million reasons per year to rationalize spreading false information that leads to more sales for Pfizer (and the deaths of many innocent people).

The other issue with this video and the dozens and dozens of others like it from Rachel and other show Hosts is here we are in September of 2022 and YouTube chooses to keep this and thousands of videos up that contain false information that leads to the death of viewers, yet they take down or shadow ban *my* videos, which contain no false or even misleading information. Ignorance and stupidity are not the cause of this deadly policy. Could promoting the Narrative, even if it is false and results in the deaths of innocent people, be their mission? It's hard to believe but it certainly appears that way.

7. https://www.youtube.com/watch?v=OrjMLONm-Bw Fauci and Walensky made dozens like this one, five months after I proved the opposite. In this video, he says: "It's as simple as black and white. You're vaccinated, you're safe. You're unvaccinated, you're at risk. Simple as that."

8. https://www.oraclefilms.com/alettertoandrewhill
Dr. Andrew Hill confesses to Dr. Tess Lawrie about having not told the truth about IVM efficacy due to

pressure from industry.

9. https://www.youtube.com/watch?v=fygh-0THA7k

Senator from Rhode Island, Jack Reed, looking very stupid while trying to make Trump look bad for not wearing masks (Senator Reed isn't wearing one either…). Neither one of them should wear a mask. They don't significantly reduce transmission of respiratory viruses. Read the literature, Senator, and you won't make yourself look stupid on national T.V. Former CDC Director Robert Redfield looks even stupider in this clip. He said, (referring to the surgical mask he is holding in his hand), "These face masks are the most important powerful public health tool we have. We have clear scientific evidence they work." Dr. Redfield, you're wrong. Please look at the literature. Look at this year's graphs. Look at this year's studies."

10 Questions Executives of Vaccine Manufacturers Must Answer Under Oath, in Senate Testimony

1. Of all the SARS-2 proteins you could have chosen to act as the antigen in your protein subunit vaccine, how could you have chosen the spike protein? You couldn't possibly have decided on a more ill-suited candidate. 1) You already knew it was toxic since data from SARS-2 infection showed that spike protein caused vascular endothelial damage and promotes clot formation, 2) this spike changes often through mutation in the RNA that codes for it (a well-known survival mechanism of this virus), 3) antibodies to the spike were likely to attack self proteins, and 4) but perhaps most inexplicable is why all four of you would pass over a an ideal candidate protein, the N-protein whose job it is to stabilize the RNA, that was well-known to have 1) not changed significantly in 17 years, 2) elicited a strong enough immune response to protect those infected back then from reinfection with a virus that is so similar to SARS-2, those infected 17 years ago are also protected against infection with SARS-2 since the N-proteins of these two viruses are similar enough to be considered identical for our purposes. Furthermore, there was no toxicity noted in the past 17 years and the antibodies elicited by it did not attack vital proteins. It was stable, did not change appreciably in a very long time, did not cause autoimmune disease, and elicited a very strong and long-lasting immune response. So please explain your thinking in choosing the worst possible candidate.

2. Were 1) blocking transmission and/or 2) prevention of severe disease and death considered as choices for primary efficacy endpoints in your trials? If not, why not?

3. What was the thinking behind your choice of primary efficacy endpoint (symptom reduction, essentially)?

4. Were you aware during the trials that the vaccines did not block transmission?

5. If not, why not? If so, why wasn't the public notified?

6. Did you not measure the vaccine's ability to block transmission because you didn't want it known (as it happened) if they could not?

7. Did your choice of the primary efficacy endpoint arise from realizing that your vaccines would impair the immune response of recipients to the degree that symptoms would be reduced, thereby making them fare better in the trials the more destructive they were?

8. Why was assessment of the effects of the vaccines on reproduction limited only to testing female rats when it was well-known that the spike protein did not interact adequately with rat ACE-2 receptors?

9. It is now known that sperm production is reduced post vaccination for five months. Early

media reports claimed reproduction was not affected. Were you aware that it was, in fact, affected in both males and females?

10. How do you explain the latest miscarriage statistics?

4 *Major Midstream Changes by the CDC, FDA, and WHO When the Data Contradicted the Narrative*

1. The Guidelines for assigning Cause of Death

See #1, "**8 *Most Important Slides of the Pandemic***"

2. The Definition of "Herd Immunity"

On November 13, 2020, The WHO inserted a new definition of herd immunity. On its Q&A page, the definition that had stood since June 9, 2020. The definition was changed from this (June 9, 2020): "Herd immunity is the indirect protection from an infectious disease that happens when a population is immune either through vaccination or immunity developed through previous infection. This means that even people who haven't been infected, or in whom an infection hasn't triggered an immune response, they are protected because people around them who are immune can act as buffers between them and an infected person. The threshold for establishing herd immunity for COVID-19 is not yet clear."This one is wrong because it is not taking into account immunity-in-place!

That definition was changed to this (on November 13, 2020): "Herd immunity is achieved by protecting people from a virus, not by exposing them to it." Then they tell you to read the Director-General's 12 October , 2020 media briefing speech for more detail. "Vaccines train our immune systems to develop antibodies, just as might happen when we are exposed to a disease but – crucially – vaccines work without making us sick. Vaccinated people are protected from getting the disease in question." This one is wrong in every way. WHO DG Tedros apparently does not understand herd immunity or what vaccines do and don't do.

3.The Definition of "Vaccine"

The CDC's definition changed from "a product that stimulates a person's immune system to produce immunity to a specific disease" to the current "a preparation that is used to stimulate the body's immune response against diseases."

They took specificity out of the definition of what constitutes a vaccine. There are some very disturbing things going on at the CDC. I hate to say this but based on their behavior over the last two-and-a-half years, I would not trust anything they say.

4. The Efficacy Threshold for approving Vaccines in Children

The FDA ignored all of the 365 COVID cases that occurred in trial participants after the first and second doses were administered, only counting the 10 that occurred after the 3rd dose. They did this because the vaccinated were getting infected more often than the placebo group. Finally, after the 3rd dose, the efficacy figure they used to approve the vaccines was based on only the 3 % of infections that occurred after the third dose.

When you include the other 97% the vaccine was only 20% effective. The threshold for approving these vaccines was set at 50% in 2020 yet they approved them anyway. There was absolutely no justification for approving these dangerous vaccines and the FDA should be seriously reprimanded for this. The members of the committee that approved them should be prosecuted criminally and exposed to civil judgments if anyone is injured by their fraud and malfeasance.

8 Visual Lies Told To the Public
(there were thousands)

1.

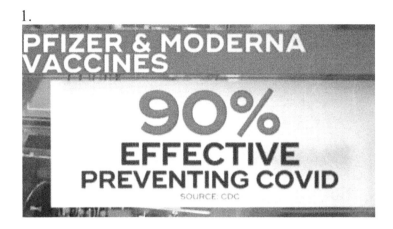

This flagrant lie was sent out by the CDC on March 29, 2021, and was repeated on local and national news outlets all over America. It was two-and-a-half months AFTER I had proved that the vaccines did not prevent one from getting COVID.

2.

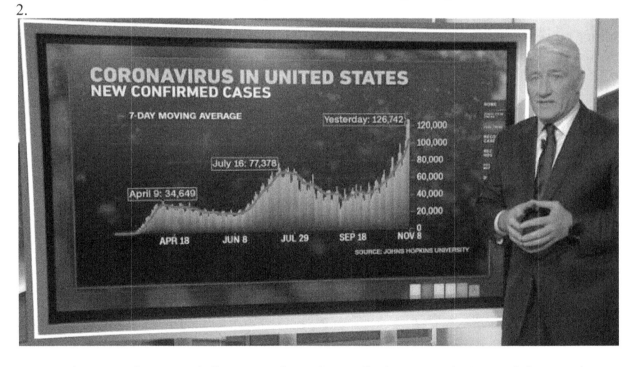

Sorry, John King. Those aren't "New, Confirmed Cases". They were designated that way because of the PCR test. That test does not look for viable virus. It looks for RNA fragments. Those fragments can still be present in the mucus of the nasopharynx up to three months after someone has recovered from the virus. Your lie exaggerates the case, hospitalization and death counts an estimated 6, 7, 8 times the actual number. This was the basis for assigning COVID-19 as the cause of death even when there was a clear alternative cause. By lying like this, you increased fear in the population which made people accept destructive and deadly policies like lockdowns, and experimental injections of which we knew nothing of their long-term side effects. As a result of this, many of those same people were severely injured, lost their life savings, their jobs and the health insurance that came with it. Many died in the following years because they were unable to afford investigations of suspicious breast lumps, screening colonoscopies, and other life-saving measures.

3.

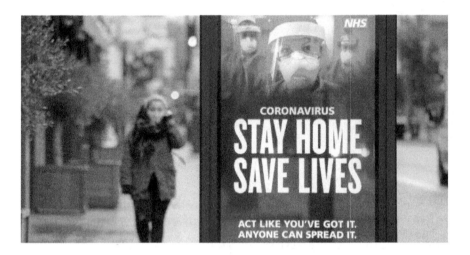

This one from over in England. Sorry, NHS. Staying home causes more people to die. You have it exactly backwards Getting outside was safer as we have been trying to tell you since the beginning. (please see slide #3 of *"9 Most Important Slides of the Pandemic."*)

4.

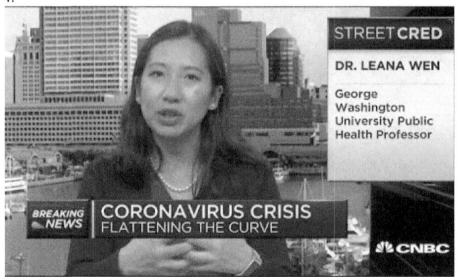

If the people in charge had listened to people who understood this, we never would have gone into lockdowns. They were the exact OPPOSITE of what we needed to do to reduce our risk. This was obvious before we went into them. But even if people couldn't understand why, all they had to do was look at any graph of cases vs. time for any country. Not only were there no flattening of any curves anywhere at any time, you couldn't even find a single case of an ascending slope decreasing. Did Dr. Leana Wen understand this? If she did, she's part-responsible for over 100 million deaths . If she didn't, she has no business putting herself up as an expert. " Street Cred"; what a joke.

5.

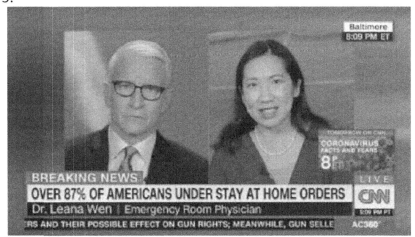

"Over 87% of Americans under stay at home orders" . These people lost their jobs, their health insurance, their life savings, and in some instances, their shelter. These people could not afford to get colonoscopies and are dying now and are dying now from metastatic colon cancer. They couldn't get their breast lumps biopsied. They are dying of metastatic breast cancer now. But not Dr. Leana Wen and Anderson Cooper. Their salaries never stopped. Leana Wen's increased by what she was making from CNN, telling lies about the "benefits" of lockdowns. This is a good example of why we should never forget who was spreading lies and what lies they were spreading in the early days of the fraud.

6.

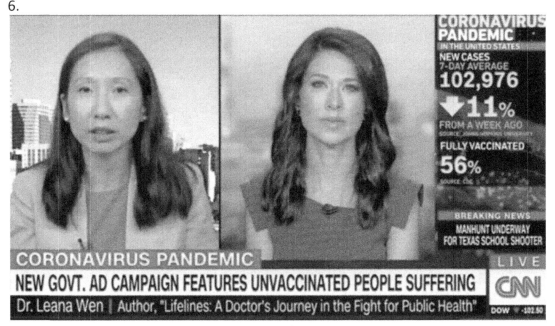

You're not allowed to have a book title like this if you're pushing lockdowns. They were the single most deadly public health policy in the history of mankind. "A Doctor's Journey in the Fight for Public Health"?? In this appearance, she's also pushing the horrible vaccines on unsuspecting people without knowing anything about the long term side effects of those vaccines. How could any doctor do something so irresponsible with the health of an entire nation?

7.

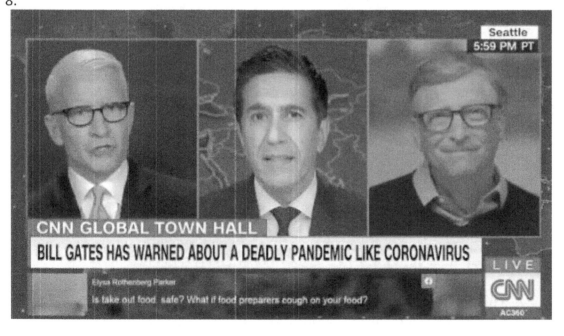

Lots of lying on this slide. They've got deaths in the US at more than one fifth of the world. That's because we exaggerated our death totals. (please see slides 7. And 9. of "**9 Most Important Slides of the Pandemic**"). Also shown is another person- a modeler from the U. of Washington- who thinks" if most wore masks", we could save half of 168,000 deaths. This person needs to read the literature and look at all of the graphs that had been produced by then and show us where mask use was correlated with the improvements he is claiming.

8.

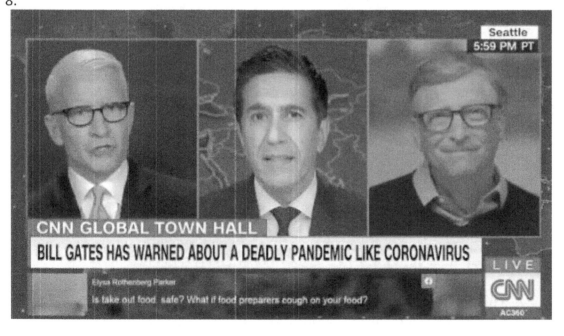

Why was Bill Gates invited onto shows like this. In February of 2020, he wrote an article in the New England Journal of Medicine making a case that COVID-19 had shown recent signs that it might be the "Pandemic of the Century". He's someone who suggested we increase our tracing in October of 2020, 10 months after the virus was in the US. For a respiratory virus... As smart as Bill is, he doesn't seem to be able to apply his considerable reasoning ability to medical issues. Some have said, he made those less-than-insightful statements on purpose; that the early fear-mongering ones were meant to increase sales of the vaccine as by this time, he had made a major investment in BioNTech. We may not ever find out. Recently, he claimed neither he nor the doctors at the Bill and Melinda Gates Foundation did not know the IFR was so low and that COVID-19 was a disease of the elderly but this is contradicted by the article mentioned above (please see slide #9 in "*9 Most important Slides of the Pandemic*")

3 Reasons Why We Can Be Sure There Was Planning Beforehand

1. All Four major vaccine makers choosing the spike protein as the antigen upon which immune systems are directed was so illogical, as to be below the lower limit of what is possible from sheer stupidity.
A) We've known for years that the spike protein changed often. It was a survival mechanism for the spike to evade antibodies from memory B cells and cell destruction compliments of CD8 and CD4 subsets of Cellular Immunity (the T-Cell side of the Adaptive Immune System) B) We knew as soon as antibodies were produced to the spike protein on the surface of the virus, that there was cross reactivity with body protein which could lead to autoimmune diseases. In fact, of all 29 proteins in SARS-2, the spike protein has the second-greatest numbers of epitopes (antibody binding sites) that were similar enough to human epitopes to cause auto-immunity. This should have eliminated the spike protein from the running as a choice to elicit even larger numbers of antibodies via the vaccines since safety is always the most important consideration. You are giving the vaccine to lots of healthy people, and you don't want to make the population sicker from the vaccine than they would have gotten from the disease.

One issue in this regard concerned the manufacturers not knowing how long the mRNA would remain viable in cells. Too long and enormous amounts of spike protein would be released, increasing the risk of auto-immune disease. Too short and you wouldn't make the number of spike proteins required to produce enough antibodies to defeat invading viruses, and C) We knew the spike protein was toxic on its own very early on in the infection. It was the spike on the virus itself that caused most of the problems that arose from getting COVID-19, for example, stroke and heart attack. The spike protein was the worst antigen candidate you could think of. The odds that any one of the four vaccine manufacturers would choose it were far less than 1 in 100. 1/100 multiplied by itself 4 times is 1 chance in 100 million. It could not have happened out of sheer stupidity on all their parts. There had to be collusion.

I remember thinking out loud when making a video in mid-2020 about how the mRNA vaccines worked and blurting out, "Why did they choose the spike protein? It's going to mutate and change its antibody binding sites (epitopes) very often." And then mumbling, "Maybe they want to sell more vaccines..."And I believe that's exactly why they chose it; so they could make more money selling the multiple vaccines that would be needed to chase all the variants that would result from the spike protein changing so often. This proves malfeasance. If a vaccine manufacturer commits this kind of fraud, malfeasance and collusion, do they still get to enjoy blanket immunity against lawsuits arising out of poor outcomes? The trial data that the FDA wanted to hide for 75 years has shown that the vaccine companies were aware of many adverse effects the vaccine manufacturers kept from the public. This should be the next huge wave of investigations and the individuals involved in withholding this information should be tried and sent to prison if found guilty. It is not enough just to impose a fine on the companies themselves. This is why this book was written- to expose the individuals behind this massive crime and make them pay their debt to society. Fines amounting to the most in history times ten would not affect these companies significantly and they would continue to engage in this criminal activity the next time around. But if individuals are held accountable and individuals are made to return their ill-gotten gains, people contemplating this kind of activity will think twice next time and probably will decline. This is the only way we can make our society better.

D) We had already checked the blood of recovered SARS patients and found out two very important things: 1) the patients were still protected from getting SARS due to memory T cells still circulating there, and 2) patients who had never been exposed to the SARS-2 virus were protected from getting infected with that virus as well. Cross reactivity, not just reactivity to the protein you were made for originally, but for a virus that arose 20 years later.

The N Protein is one stable protein and was clearly the best choice by a huge margin. The spike protein was the worst. The chance that all of the scientists at all four Companies manufacturing vaccines could have made the same mistake is almost zero. Given that there are many proteins in the virus that were better choices than the spike protein and one sitting right in front of them with a 17 year track record of stability, no known autoimmune cross-reactivity, and no known toxicity, there is about a one in 100 chance a team of scientists set with the task of choosing the best candidate for the vaccine could have chosen the spike protein, a horrible candidate that failed on every measure. Now consider that the teams of all four vaccine makers came up with the same idiotic choice.

Knowing these characteristics of the spike, and given that we already had a perfect candidate waiting in the wings, the chance is almost zero that they didn't commit the crime of collusion. And they did it knowing the spike proteins would change frequently and the public would need to be protected with a new vaccine more than once a year (and the more money they would make). Plus, why not put two mRNA sequences in the lipid nanoparticles that make up the vaccine? I don't know some of the technical aspects of adding another piece of genetic material but I doubt it's a problem because there is not one mRNA molecule in a lipid nanoparticle (LNP), there are up to 200, depending on the size of the LNP.

Remember one final thing about the choice of the spike protein. They all had to choose it. If any of the four companies had chosen a better protein's genomic sequence to put into their mRNA vaccine, the public would have noticed very early on that that was the superior vaccine. They would have used that one exclusively and none of the companies would have made the enormous amount of money they have made off of convincing the public they needed to get booster after booster.

The vaccines have performed so poorly that it would be fair to say the only result of this supposed effort to protect the public from a virus of very limited virulence was to transfer enormous sums of money- some say $3.8 trillion- from the general public to a few thousand individuals. The few thousand including major social media stockholders, those with major ownership in vaccine companies and those whose small companies received large grants to produce vaccines, producers of PPE such as masks, gowns, face shields, etc., and people who developed tests, testing equipment and testing supplies, etc.

2. The fake videos of people foaming at the mouth and collapsing dead on the streets of Wuhan. These videos were meant to scare Americans and it worked. Just take a look at the comments under this video: https://www.youtube.com/watch?v=Uf4-Vzf1CyM. Those from two years ago show that people thought the video was legit. They were genuinely scared by what they saw. Those from one year ago are joking about how fake it looks. It really does look fake to anyone caring to look closely. The falling people either land on cushions placed out of view or they stick out their hands to cushion the fall. People who really pass out don't do that. Their heads hit the basketball court or the ground so hard, they are difficult to watch as in this video: https://www.youtube.com/watch?v=1Ni5l96kS-Q . It is heartbreaking to watch it. We have not seen a single person collapsing like this from COVID but we have seen dozens and dozens do so after the vaccines. Many believe it is because of myocarditis caused by the vaccines, sudden fatal heart attacks or strokes. Young male athletes in the target age group are collapsing and dying on the soccer pitch and basketball court, primarily. If you look at the number who "dropped dead" on the pitch in past seasons and compare it to what has happened since these athletes were required to get the vaccine, you will be shocked. The ratio is about 20 to 1, depending on the league. The young men, of course, are among the best conditioned athletes in the world.

The fake videos definitely served their purpose. China wanted to scare the rest of the world into accepting lockdowns that the Chinese authorities encouraged other governments to use.

The purposeful release to the world of pictures of a city-wide fountain party that took place in Wuhan a few months after their very severe lockdowns ended.

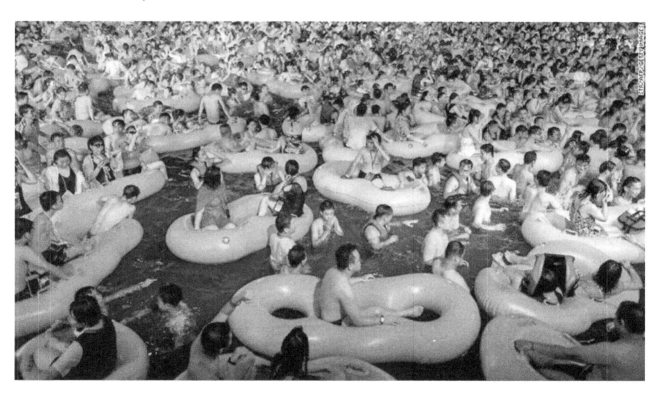

Even if you believe lockdowns flatten the curve, you don't believe lockdowns prevent you from getting infected in the future. No one in their right mind would hold a city-wide party in the middle of a pandemic caused by a virus transmitted by respiratory aerosols.

The Chinese authorities were trying to show the world how well the lockdowns worked and our stupid politicians fell for it. They played us like a fiddle. Since they didn't close their factories, worldwide shipping routes adjusted to pick up goods from China and their GDP rose 3.5% in 2020 while those of Europe fell by the high single digits.

3. Peter Daszak and his team in the bat caves of Yunnan province, injecting free-flying bats identified to carry high spillover risk SARS coronaviruses, with novel chimeric polyvalent recombinant spike proteins (like those present on SARS-2) while exposing them to aerosolized agents designed to boost their immune systems in an effort to down-regulate viral replication, all with the ultimate goal of developing vaccine candidates.

They will say they did all this with the goal to be ready with vaccines in the event that one of these viruses jumped the species barrier from bats to humans via natural zoonotic spillover. But that is almost too reckless to be believed, to create a super virus, capable of killing hundreds of millions of people, if not billions, just so you could experiment with different vaccines in the hopes of developing one that could ward off such a virus, if one day, it appeared. It's just too dangerous. The chance of any particular virus appearing and being infectious in humans is almost zero.

Peter Daszak explained how he was doing this in a 2018 proposal to D.A.R.P.A., submitted with the purpose of being awarded a grant to continue the practice I've described above. D.A.R.P.A. rejected his proposal as too dangerous but he got his money. Anthony Fauci stepped in to provide the funding. Daszak wasn't just proposing how he would do these things. In a November 2019 tweet, he lists these things as something he had already done.

They were planning to reverse engineer spike proteins and insert them onto SARS coronavirus *backbones* instead of SARS coronaviruses themselves, using a nice little loophole someone created for them, to skirt the laws against gain of function research, and inject them into humanized mice to see if the mice develop SARS-like illnesses. Humanized mice are mice that have had their ACE-2 receptors changed to human ACE-2 receptors to find out if the viruses injected into the mice would be able to get into human cells, a nice little trick Ralph Baric developed about ten years ago. In the subsequent years, he shipped a bunch of these mice off to Dr. Shi at the Wuhan Institute of virology. That alone should put Ralph Baric in chains for a very long time. It's no different than if an engineer at Lockheed-Martin sent a critical part of our latest fighter jet- a part they couldn't quite get right- to a fellow engineer working on fighter jets in China- not for military purposes, mind you. Crop dusting?

Daszak, Baric, Shi and others had been doing this stuff for years- at least since 2013 when the miners cleaning guano out of a mine in Mojiang, Yunnan province got infected with a virus they could never identify and later fell ill and died. That alone is questionable. Was that part of the fear campaign? Daszak's tweets and video-taped interviews provide a roadmap to every milestone they achieved. If you think I'm exaggerating the seriousness of this kind of reckless behavior, just look at where we are in the world today.

The tweet below, along with the accumulated knowledge listed above and the five-year NIH grant starting in 2014, prove that Daszak and the Wuhan Institute of Virology, to which he subcontracted part of the work, were engaged in gain of function research during the time it was banned. Dr. Fauci has been denying this in Senate testimony all year and he and Dr. Francis Collins have been leading the call to label anyone, such as myself and many others, who dare to look into this, "conspiracy theorists". Please note the date of this tweet: November 21, 2019.

Peter Daszak @PeterDaszak · Nov 21, 2019

Not true - we've made great progress with bat
SARS-related CoVs, ID'ing >50 novel strains,
sequencing spike protein genes, ID'ing ones that
bind to human cells, using recombinant
viruses/humanized mice to see SARS-like signs,
and showing some don't respond to MAbs,
vaccines... twitter.com/arambaut/statu...

Show this thread

Undergraduate Majors of 21 Heroes and Villains

1. Anthony Fauci, M.D., The Classics, College of the Holy Cross
2. Deborah Birx, M.D., Chemistry/Pre-med, Houghton University
3. Peter Daszak, PhD, Zoology, Bangor University
4. Andrew Cuomo - unknown, Fordham University
5. Ngozi Ezike, M.D., Chemistry, Harvard College
6. Norman Fenton, PhD- Mathematics, London School of Economics
7. Scott Jensen, M.D.- Physiology, University of Minnesota
8. Jay Bhattacharya, M.D., PhD- economics, Stanford
9. Francis Collins, M.D., PhD- Chemistry, University of Virginia
10. Alex Berenson- History/Economics, Yale
11. Rochelle Wallensky, M.D., Biochem./Molecular Biology, Washington University in St. Louis
12. Anders Tegnell , M.D. Medicine, Lund University
13. Sundar Pichai- Metalurgical Engineering, Indian Inst. Of Tech-Kharagpur
14. Martin Kulldorff, PhD, Mathematical statistics, Umea University
15. Sanjay Gupta, M.D.-Biomedical Sciences, University of Michigan
16. Mark Zuckerberg- Psychology/Comp. Sci., left after two years, Harvard College
17. Bill Gates- Pre-law, left after two years, Harvard College
18. Susan Wojcicki - History and Literature, Harvard College
19. Steve Kirsch- Electrical Engineering and Computer Science, M.I.T.
20. Michael Levitt, PhD- Physics, King's College, London
21. Sunetra Gupta, PhD- Biology, Princeton

1 Major Error made by the COVID-19 Vaccine Trial Designers

Fertility testing was only done for females and the testing was done in an inappropriate animal model. They used rats.

The receptors on the cells of rats bind the COVID-19 spike with less affinity than human receptors. The binding is so weak in rats they don't even get the disease we have come to know as COVID-19 when infected with the SARS-2 virus. The consequence of this is that the rat model is unable to reveal toxicities as readily as a human model (or in the general public after the vaccines are released). Here's what we learned from a recent study:

Sperm concentration was reduced by 15.4% and there were 22.1% fewer motile spermatozoa per ejaculate. Both of these findings are troubling because the name of the game in reproduction from the male end is having an abundance of motile, vigorous fast-swimming sperm.

The test subjects in this study had received two doses of the Pfizer-BioNTech only and the effects lasted around six months. If these young men continue to take boosters every six months or so, they may never reach normality. Furthermore, we don't know whether the damage will be cumulative or affect reproduction in some other way over the long run. Perhaps it is not surprising that 2022 birth rates are down from 15-30% in countries all around the world. Despite all of this, Pfizer notified the public that the vaccines seemed to have no impact on fertility.

6 Things You Can Do to Reduce Your Risk of Getting COVID-19 and Have a Milder Illness If You Do Get Infected

The principle here is to reduce the concentration of virus particles as much as possible and optimize your health and vitamin D level so if you do get infected, you'll have an easier go of it.

1. Spend time out of doors

2. Increase the ventilation in every room of your house. Open windows on both sides of your house, weather permitting. You want to make your house as much like the outdoors as possible. Houses with closed windows and doors are filled with stagnant air. Stay away from them as much as possible. Open the windows when you're sleeping.

3. Avoid sick people It's obvious, sure, because it works. The Narrative promoters had us avoid ALL people (with lockdowns, social distancing, etc.). This was not helpful and caused a lot of harm. People are very good at recognizing sick people coming toward them on the street and crossing to the other side to avoid them. We developed this skill because, before antibiotics, getting sick could easily mean death. We need to rekindle those skills.

4. Exercise, eat healthy, and lose weight. Being fit is even more important in times like these. Toward this end, I wrote a book explaining how to slim down to your weight (achieved when you reached your maximum height, around late high school or college age). I understand that it is even harder to do this when you are stuck at home and parks and athletic facilities are closed. Some people get bored being stuck at home all day and night. It's almost as if there's nothing to do but eat and drink and watch television. The book is called "The No Willpower Diet: How to Slim Down to Your Ideal Weight Without Ever Being Hungry". I figured out the system while analyzing alternative energy sources proposed to combat climate change. I tried it on 15 friends, all of whom had a weight problem, including me! Everyone lost over 30 pounds and I lost 56. I went from 248 pounds to 192 in four months, losing between 1/3 to ½ pound a day until I stopped losing. I never got hungry (that's why I called it the No

Willpower Diet…) After about two weeks, my taste buds changed to where I lost interest in the unhealthy foods I used to eat. Friends of mine whose bellies had devolved into the middle-age paunch, regained their washboard abdomens. My girlfriend, who, at 5'4" always weighs between 92 and 95 pounds, ate the same food as me and her weight didn't change because she was already at her ideal weight. She's the one on the cover of The No Willpower Diet at heroesandvillainsbooks.com.

5. Get your Vitamin D Level in Order and don't forget zinc. I'd like you to get your vitamin D level to around 50 ng/ml. Something magical happens at 30 ng/ml and it's tempting to think you are protected if you get your level above 30 but to be on the safe side, get it up to 50 ng/ml. 30 ng/ml is used in all the studies because it is an inflection point. Above 30 ng/ml, only about 5% of the patients die. Between 20 and 30, though, and we see about 90% dying and below 20 ng/ml, almost everyone dies. Here is a long video I made a few years ago. I explain everything you need to know about vitamin D.

https://www.youtube.com/watch?v=BLUcF2itt6c&t=3584s

Let me end with a few very important facts about vitamin D levels. 1. Most people have levels below 30, 2. 90 % of your active form of vitamin D is converted from cholesterol in your skin, so get out in the sun. A good 30 minutes a day with the sun baking your back will help you maintain your vitamin D level but it needs to be checked and monitored. 3. If you live above the 35th parallel (or below it in the southern hemisphere)., you cannot get adequate sun in the winter because it comes in at too acute an angle. This means that you're going to need supplements in the winter. The area above the 35th parallel includes all of Europe and about 90% of the US. Please get your vitamin D level above 50 ng/ml. It is critical to your health for many reasons, not just to fend off COVID-19.

Get a zinc supplement and take it. Around 50mg per day should be adequate.

6. Prophylax with Ivermectin or Hydroxychloroquine. More and more studies are coming out now that show these two medicines are effective in preventing and treating COVID-19. Choose based on which one is shown to be more effective against the variant in question. Not everyone has to take them but you should as a preventative if you're in a high risk group or high risk situation and you should definitely start them immediately upon noticing symptoms. They offer significant benefits but it's not 100%. Vicious propaganda campaigns were waged against them because if they had been allowed on the market, the vaccines wouldn't have been able to get emergency use authorization. Many tens of billions of dollars were at stake for the vaccine makers and they weren't going to let the public's health get in the way.

8 Deeply Disturbing Letters, Memos or Emails

1. From Peter Daszak to Anthony Fauci on April 18, 2020
   Thanking each other for lying to the public…

From:	Fauci, Anthony (NIH/NIAID) [E]
Sent:	Sun, 19 Apr 2020 03:29:42 +0000
To:	Peter Daszak
Subject:	RE: Thank you for your public comments re COVID-19's origins

Peter:

Many thanks for your kind note.

Best regards,

Tony

From: Peter Daszak [(b) (6)]
Sent: Saturday, April 18, 2020 9:43 PM
To: Morens, David (NIH/NIAID) [E] [(b) (6)]; Fauci, Anthony (NIH/NIAID) [E]
[(b) (6) >
Cc: Stemmy, Erik (NIH/NIAID) [E] [(b) (6) >; Erbelding, Emily (NIH/NIAID) [E]
[(b) (6) >; Aleksei Chmura [(b) (6)]
Subject: Thank you for your public comments re COVID-19's origins
Importance: High

Tony (cc'ing David so that you might pass this on to Tony once he has a spare second)

As the PI of the R01 grant publicly targeted by Fox News reporters at the Presidential press briefing last night, I just wanted to say a personal thankyou on behalf of our staff and collaborators, for publicly standing up and stating that the scientific evidence supports a natural origin for COVID-19 from a bat-to-human spillover, not a lab release from the Wuhan Institute of Virology.

(b) (7)(A)

From my perspective, your comments are brave, and coming from your trusted voice, will help dispel the myths being spun around the virus' origins.

2. From Francis Collins to Anthony Fauci and Cliff Lane on October 8, 2020. (Note: The Great Barrington Declaration was posted on October 5, 2020)
   "A quick and devastating take down of its premises". What a disaster Dr. Collins created for himself with this email.

From: Collins, Francis (NIH/OD) [E]   (b) (6)
Sent: Thursday, October 8, 2020 2:31 PM
To: Fauci, Anthony (NIH/NIAID) [E]   (b) (6); Lane, Cliff (NIH/NIAID) [E]
     (b) (6)
Cc: Tabak, Lawrence (NIH/OD) [E]   (b) (6)
Subject: Great Barrington Declaration

Hi Tony and Cliff,

See https://gbdeclaration.org/ This proposal from the three fringe epidemiologists who met with the Secretary seems to be getting a lot of attention – and even a co-signature from Nobel Prize winner Mike Leavitt at Stanford. There needs to be a quick and devastating published take down of its premises. I don't see anything like that on line yet – is it underway?

Francis

3. From Mark Zuckerberg (through Courtney Billet) to Anthony Fauci on March 16, 2020

What Deal Did Mark Zuckerberg offer Dr. Fauci on March 16, 2020 that needed to be redacted? All of the people copied on these emails should be brought in for questioning under oath. What are our Senators and Congressmen and women doing? They haven't even brought in Ralph Baric and Peter Daszak in yet!

From: Fauci, Anthony (NIH/NIAID) [E]
Sent: Tue, 17 Mar 2020 00:23 16 +0000
To: Billet, Courtney (NIH/NIAID) [E]
Cc: Folkers, Greg (NIH/NIAID) [E];Conrad, Patricia (NIH/NIAID) [E];Stover, Kathy (NIH/NIAID) [E],Routh, Jennifer (NIH/NIAID) [E]
Subject: RE: offer from Mark Zuckerberg

I will write to or call Mark and tell him that I am interested in doing this. I will then tell him that you will get for him the name of the USG point of contact. I agree it should be Bill Hall who could then turf to the White House Comms if he wishes

From: Billet, Courtney (NIH/NIAID) [E]   (b) (6)>
Sent: Monday, March 16, 2020 6.53 PM
To: Fauci, Anthony (NIH/NIAID) [E] <   (b) (6)>
Cc: Folkers, Greg (NIH/NIAID) [E]   (b) (6); Conrad, Patricia (NIH/NIAID) [E]
     (b) (6); Stover, Kathy (NIH/NIAID) [E]   (b) (6)>; Routh, Jennifer (NIH/NIAID) [E]   (b) (6) >
Subject: ASF: offer from Mark Zuckerberg

Per email below, Mark Zuckerberg has extended a few offers to do videos with you that we would be happy to seek clearance on for you to do, if you are amenable. These would have the weight and impact of television – really, more so. Please advise if you want to do and we will seek clearance with VP office and work with Patty to sort out the logistics.

But an even bigger deal is his offer   (b) (4)
     The sooner we get that offer up the food-chain the better. I gave Bill Hall a heads-up about this opportunity and he is standing by to discuss this with HHS and WH comms, but I didn't want him to do anything without you being aware of the offer. Is it OK if I hand this aspect off to Bill to determine who the best point of contact would be so the Administration can take advantage of this offer, soonest?

Do you plan to call MZ? His cell number is in his message below.

145

From: Fauci, Anthony (NIH/NIAID) [E]
Sent: Sat, 1 Feb 2020 18:43:31 +0000
To: Kristian G. Andersen
Subject: RE: FW: Science: Mining coronavirus genomes for clues to the outbreak's origins

Thanks, Kristian.   Talk soon on the call.

From: Kristian G. Andersen [(b) (6) >
Sent: Friday, January 31, 2020 10:32 PM
To: Fauci, Anthony (NIH/NIAID) [E][(b) (6)
Cc: Jeremy Farrar [(b) (6) >
Subject: Re: FW: Science: Mining coronavirus genomes for clues to the outbreak's origins

Hi Tony,

Thanks for sharing. Yes, I saw this earlier today and both Eddie and myself are actually quoted in it. It's a great article, but the problem is that our phylogenetic analyses aren't able to answer whether the sequences are unusual at individual residues, except if they are completely off. On a phylogenetic tree the virus looks totally normal and the close clustering with bats suggest that bats serve as the reservoir. The unusual features of the virus make up a really small part of the genome (<0.1%) so one has to look really closely at all the sequences to see that some of the features (potentially) look engineered.

We have a good team lined up to look very critically at this, so we should know much more at the end of the weekend. I should mention that after discussions earlier today, Eddie, Bob, Mike, and myself all find the genome inconsistent with expectations from evolutionary theory. But we have to look at this much more closely and there are still further analyses to be done, so those opinions could still change.

Best,
Kristian

On Fri, Jan 31, 2020 at 18:47 Fauci, Anthony (NIH/NIAID) [E] [(b) (6) > wrote:

> Jeremy/Kristian:
>   This just came out today.   You may have seen it.   If not, it is of interest to the current
> discussion.
>   Best,
>   Tony

Within 2 days of this email, and a secret teleconference Kristian Andersen, Robert Garry, Ian Lipkin, Edward Homes and Andrew Rambaut authored a paper entitled "The Proximal Origin of SARS-CoV-2" which pushed the natural origin theory for SARS-2. They had earlier told Fauci that the genome of the virus looked engineered (shown above).

They decided to write the paper during or shortly after the teleconference and even had the first draft finished the same day as the teleconference. In the next two years, some shared $50 million of funding from Fauci. This is outright fraud- to be awarding taxpayer-funded grants to these people based on doing a favor for the corrupt leader, instead of the merits of their proposals.

What are congressmen and Senators waiting for? Bring these people in for questioning!

4 Groups Responsible for Allowing Misery, Destruction, and Death in Victoria, Australia

Australia/New Zealand was the region of the world where government officials abused their residents most aggressively. Victoria, Australia, under Daniel Andrews, was the poster child. From the beginning, they locked down and locked down hard; the exact opposite of what they should have done. The effect on peoples' civil liberties and children's education was devastating. Transgressions, even protests, were contained as brutally as any you might see in old film clips of the most sadistic regimes in history. I've never seen so many frail people being beaten with police batons in my life. Old ladies were hit with batons and went down to the pavement. When they looked up policemen sprayed them point-blank in the eyes with mace. When the vaccines became available, the officials there moved just as aggressively, again with devastating consequences.

1. Members of the Victoria Police Force who did not resign within days of the government's sadistic orders to enforce (worthless) lockdowns, border closures and the government's violent reaction to peaceful protests by the citizens of Victoria.

2. Supporters of "Stand with Dan"

3. The Medical Doctors of Australia Where were those of you who understood the science behind COVID-19 and the vaccines? It was YOUR responsibility to step up and stop the violent madness that was being inflicted on your fellow citizens at the hands of the political class and police. If you did not understand the science, you should have gotten on the internet and listened to those of us in other countries who did.

4. The men of Australia. Band together and never ever let this sort of thing happen again. The police were beating elderly women with clubs. Take a flamethrower to the place if you have to.

43 Idiotic Quotes Surrounding the Pandemic

1. WHO Director-General Tedros: "COVID-19 is a new virus and nobody has immunity to it." The Director-General of the World Health Organization doesn't understand basic immunology. That's a recipe for billions wasted (or more likely stolen) per year. Get someone in there who knows something.

2. Dr. Francis Collins (Director of the NIH): "Masks prevent the spread of the virus." This person is in charge of our National Institutes of health. The degree of stupidity of these people is utterly mindboggling.

3. William Haseltine, PhD: "Herd immunity is another word for mass murder." This person is not an M.D. but he should know that herd immunity is a good thing. "Mass Murder"?

4. William Haseltine, PhD: "If the virus is allowed to spread, we are looking at two to six million Americans dead, not just this year but every year." This is beyond stupid.

5. Marty Makary, M.D. on June 15, 2020 " … and we can have those debates (of mask effectiveness). We have a country of opinions and we need to put those opinions aside. Whatever the effectiveness of the mask is, whether it's a 30% mitigation or a 60% mitigation in reducing the velocity of transmission, it's one of the few tools we have. Look at Asia, look at Europe. Look at many of the states in the northern United States. They have been able to manage the infection after initial spikes and surges because of universal masking."

All of this is wrong. The literature shows meta analyses of 72 years of randomized, controlled trials. In not one, did the use of masks to control the spread of influenza, make a significant difference in transmission. This is not Monday morning quarterbacking. I had been trying to make people understand this three months earlier, since March of 2020.

Dr. Makary also stated that universal masking was the reason why cases came down and stayed down in northern states "after initial spikes and surges". That's also false. Once you realize masks don't do anything significant to reduce transmission, you stop attributing reductions in cases, hospitalizations, and deaths to masks. All you have to do is plot mask usage by percent of the population vs. time and cases vs. time on the same graph. You'll see there's no correlation. Cases came down because the virus's

R-value went below 1; the virus was having trouble finding anyone else to spread to after wreaking havoc on some parts of the northeast, such as New Your City. In fact, when Connecticut imposed fines for not wearing masks, cases went straight up and states who did not mandate mask wearing did slightly better than their neighbors who did. Look at North Dakota and South Dakota Finally, the beginning of the quote. To suggest that "we should put peoples' opinions aside" frankly that are more reasoned on the question of mask use is what got us into trouble in the first place. Censors, such as the CEOs at YouTube, Facebook and Twitter silenced people who understood this virus and disease while letting others spew utter nonsense. A lot of people lost their life savings and livelihoods over this. Some lost their lives.

6. Bill Gates: "If a country does what Australia did, the world could prevent the next pandemic."

7. Bill Gates: (from an article dated October 14, 2020) "Right now, testing, contract tracing- we're doing among the worst of any country." Contract tracing? Really, Bill? For a virus transmitted by aerosols, with virus particles that can stay in the air for days? For a virus that has been in the U.S. for almost a year? Why don't you explain to everyone how you'll be able to tell from whom an infected person got the virus. It was too late for contact tracing in January. How could you not understand something this simple?

8. Celine Gounder, M.D.: "It's a slam dunk in favor of the COVID vaccines" (referring to the 6 month to 5 year age group).

9. Johns Hopkins.com: "Both influenza and SARS-2 can be prevented by mask-wearing, frequent and thorough hand washing, coughing into the crook of your elbow".

10. Dr. Eric Rubin (sits on the FDA's VRBPAC):"We're never going to learn about how safe this vaccine is unless we start giving it." Rubin's quote is correct because, God knows, they didn't find out during the trials. But nobody in their right mind would give a vaccine to a group of people who have a miniscule chance of a severe outcome from the disease. On top of that, these vaccines do not prevent you from getting or transmitting the virus- as near to a worthless product as you can get.

11. British PM Boris Johnson: "This is the biggest challenge this country has faced since the war." Not until you instituted idiotic policies to combat it!

12. A. Odysseus Patrick: "Australia has almost eliminated the coronavirus- by putting faith in science." No. Australian authorities did the opposite of what should be done. They had their people stay indoors in stagnant air where the density of virus particles per volume of air is much greater than outside.

13. Adam Van Koeverden: "F**k you." (on social media) to an unvaccinated lady who criticized the government's ongoing vaccine mandates. Van Koeverden is a Liberal MP and Parliamentary Secretary to the Minister of Health and the Minister of Sport.

14. Klaus Schwab, WEF "Nobody will be safe if not everybody is vaccinated." No. No, no, no.

15. Celine Gounder, M.D.: "My little sister Stephanie can't wait to get her two-and-a-half-year-old daughter, Adele, vaccinated."

16. Vinay Prasad:, M.D., MPH: "You will eventually get Covid many times in your life. By now, you already got the vax or had it". (Sentence one: No. Some people will not get it. Immunity-in-place is present in at least one third of the population. That's 120 million people. Some of them might start getting it if the virus changes enough in the region of cross-reactivity they are presently benefitting from. Sentence two: No. It's not either/or. The vaccine does not prevent you from getting it.)

17. Soren Brostrom Director of the National Board of Health, Denmark: "At the time, July of 2021, it was said that the vaccinations were not predominantly for the children's own sake, but to ensure epidemic control in Denmark. It was not a mistake to vaccinate them." He's wrong. It was a huge mistake to vaccinate children in July of 2021. By then, 7 months had passed since I proved that the vaccines did not prevent transmission. He should have known that it wouldn't do anything to "ensure epidemic control".

These people are incredibly lazy, incredibly dumb, just don't care, or are getting bribes in some form to commit these atrocities.

18. A TIME Magazine tweet states, "You could have Long COVID and not even know it." Of course this means that half of us could have "long flu" from an old bout with seasonal influenza and not know it. It's just more nonsensical gibberish meant to scare, extend, and make more out of this thing than there really is. Long COVID is also meant to cover for complications of the vaccines.

19. n, M.D., MSc in February, 2022: "People who are unvaccinated have about 20 times the risk of dying of COVID and there's no question that these vaccines are effective and I would urge everybody to get vaccinated and get boosted when it's recommended."

20. Vinay Prasad, M.D., MPH on July 1, 2022: "Vaccines and weight loss are all we can do to lower our risk of getting very sick from COVID." How could someone as sophisticated and knowledgeable as Dr. Prasad not know about the benefits of getting one's vitamin D in order? Zinc, anyone? Exercise, fresh air? A healthy diet? The list goes on.

21. Megan Ranney, M.D., MPH: "I think that in a few months, we are going to be able to say with certainty that these vaccines not only protect you, they also protect those around you."

22. Vinay Prasad, M.D., MPH: "Every person on earth will get COVID 19 in the short term". No. Some people have immunity-in-place. Why did some nursing home residents not get it? Why were the 23 people they found who had survived SARS-1 also protected against SARS-2 17 years later? The answer is that they had immunity-in-place due to their clonal memory for the N-protein also protecting them from getting SARS-2.

23. Dr. Marion F. Gruber, Dr. Philip Krause, Paul Offit, M.D.: "The only strategy that will defeat the coronavirus is vaccinating the unvaccinated, wherever they live."

24. Deborah Birx, M.D.: "This is one of the most highly-effective vaccines we have in our infectious disease arsenal. And so that's why I'm very enthusiastic about the vaccine", on an ABC podcast. Birx also said, in an interview with Neil Cavuto on FOX, "I knew these vaccines were not going to protect against infection." I believe Dr. Birx is not telling the truth when she says this because on December 15, 2020 one day before the vaccines were released to the public, she said, "To truly achieve herd immunity, it's going to take through the summer and potentially even into the fall. That's getting 70-80% of Americans immunized." If the vaccines don't block transmission, they don't do anything to help us reach herd immunity. So Birx is not telling the truth when she said recently, "I knew these vaccines were not going to protect against infection."

25. Jacinda Arden, Prime Minister of New Zealand: "People who are vaccinated won't get sick and won't die:" (she said this in late 2021 after hundreds of thousands of vaccinated people had died of COVID-19, from complications of the vaccines, and from other causes.

26. Paul Offit, M.D.: "The mask. It's such an important tool. It's such a powerful tool."

27. China Medical to the WHO to the public (early January): "SARS-2 does not transmit person-to-person."

28. WHO Director-General Tedros: "Vaccinated people are protected from getting the disease in question."

29. The WHO: "The main modes of transmission of the virus are by water droplets expelled by coughing, sneezing and singing."

30. Rochelle Walensky, M.D., CDC Director: "This is a pandemic of the unvaccinated." (Months after it clearly was not)

31. Justin Trudeau, Prime minister of Canada: "If you don't want to get vaccinated, that's your choice. But don't think you can get on a plane or a train beside vaccinated people and put them at risk!" Does he realize he just told the Canadian people the vaccine doesn't protect them?

32. Dr. Bonnie Henry: "There is no [lower] limit to the age at which somebody can consent to medical treatment and that includes immunization so you don't need to have a parent's consent, you don't need to have a signed consent form".

33. Deborah Birx, M.D.: "We have worked to find a path that is least destructive to the economy".

34. Vinay Prasad, M.D., MPH: "Over the next few years, COVID-19 will engulf everyone on Earth. Over the next few decades, it will engulf everyone many times over." No, because some people have immunity-in-place due to a protein that will not change during those times or will get the disease once and acquire clonal expansion and memory to a protein that does not change in those time frames.

35. Rachel Maddow (March 21, 2021): "The virus stops with every vaccinated person. A vaccinated person gets exposed to the virus, the virus does not infect them. The virus cannot then use that person to go anywhere else. It cannot use a vaccinated person as a host to get other people."

36. Dr. F. Perry Wilson, M.D.: "Vaccines have performed better in this pandemic than we had any right to hope for".

37. Deborah Birx, M.D.: "Without masks and social distancing in public and homes, we end up with twice as many deaths."

38. Jen Psaki: "We don't know" (whether COVID-19 harms older people more than younger people). Old people die at a ratio of 1,000 to 1 to 10,000 to 1, depending on the point at which one considers someone to be old. How could she make a statement like that, given what we've known from the beginning?

39. Peter Hotez, M.D., PhD: "Teachers will be terrified, and appropriately so, about going back to work". It was never appropriate for teachers to be terrified about going back to work. This was never the case, not even close.

40. Rachel Maddow and Rochelle Walensky, M.D., MPH MADDOW:"We need to vaccinate as many people as possible as fast as possible, really, as suddenly as possible, to prevent the emergence and circulation of the variants. Is that fair?" WALENSKY: "You are exactly right." Sorry, but this has got to be one of the stupidest things I have heard the entire pandemic. Dear Dr. Walensky: THE VACCINES DO NOT BLOCK TRANSMISSION OF THE VIRUS! I proved it in mid-January, 2021.

You are the CDC Director. How could you not know something that important about the vaccines? What is worse, you kept saying the vaccine could not be transmitted from person to person until July at least. That was a full six months after I had proved the opposite. The general medical community started to pick up on this in April and you still didn't have it by July.

Rachel Maddow, who understandably doesn't know anything about the subject, said we needed to give the vaccines as quickly as possible to as many people to prevent the emergence of new variants. IT IS EXACTLY THE OPPOSITE. Giving vaccines that do not block transmission during an active pandemic is the very reason why strong variants emerge. The vaccines provide selective pressure. And Walensky said, "You are exactly right." This video was recorded from an interview that took place on MSNBC TV. It was posted on YouTube. Wojcicki allowed this 100% false information to stay up for a year-and-a half and counting while they took down some of my videos within minutes, videos that had no false or misleading statements on them. Here's the video: https://www.youtube.com/watch?v=fcTCwMqI5Z0 Look at the expression on Dr. Walensky's face as she tells these lies. Has withholding data from the public and disseminating false information gotten to her conscience?)

41. Robert Redfield, M.D., Former CDC Director: "These face masks are the most important public health tool we have. We have clear scientific evidence they work."
No they aren't, and No you don't, Dr. Redfield.
42. Ashish Jha, M.D., MPH: "Ivermectin is great as a dewormer in horses. It does not work for COVID. We all wish it did. It doesn't. But thankfully we have drugs that do. Like Paxlovid. So if you get COVID — skip the Ivermectin and get a medicine that works." Look at the literature, Dr. Jha.
43. Anthony Fauci, M.D. (June 22, 2021 on MSNBC): "It's as simple as black and white. You're vaccinated, you're safe. You're unvaccinated, you're at risk. Simple as that."
44. Bill Gates: "Normalcy only returns when we have largely vaccinated the entire global population." Vith a vaccine that doesn't block transmission and causes more death than it prevents?? The stupidity is mind-boggling.
45. Monica Ghandi, M.D.: "Masks were important until we got to a vaccine." No . Neither masks nor vaccines block transmission.
46.

15 *COVID Debates I'd Pay to See*

1. Judy Mikovits vs. Anthony Fauci
2. Sunetra Gupta vs. Deborah Birx
3. Martin Kulldorff vs. Rochelle Walensky
4. Steve Kirsch vs. Bill Gates
5. John Lee vs. Jeremy Farrar
6. Norman Fenton vs. Jason Abaluck
7. Mike Yeadon vs. Albert Bourla
8. Jay Bhattacharya vs. Randi Weingarten
9. Byram Bridle vs. Theresa Tam
10. Scott Atlas vs. Sanjay Gupta
11. Peter McCullough vs. Eric Topol
12. Robert Malone vs. Stephan Bancel
13. Ivor Cummins vs. Neil Ferguson
14. Steven Quay vs. Kristian Anderson
15. Tom Cotton vs. Justin Trudeau
16. Steven Quay vs. Robert Garry

Part 2

Chapter 1

Author's note: Dr. Michael Yeadon kindly contributed the final two chapters to this book when I asked him for only a simple list. I couldn't find anything we disagreed on as far as the medical aspects of this were concerned. You will learn , in a few pages, that our discussion led to an important discovery that had stumped many scientists looking into this. I have to give credit to Dr. Steven Quay as well who shared some information with me in a podcast that I used to resolve the problem. It's a very subtle and fascinating "tell" in the viral genome that you will learn about soon. It is also the subject of a disagreement I had with Dr. Bhattacharya during our 24 hours of video discussions; it's a little piece of the SARS-2 genome and it makes possible an exception for something that should not be able to happen according to my reasoning from first principles.

How Much of the COVID-19 Narrative Was True? –Michael Yeadon, PhD

It is contended that all the main narrative points about the virus are lies. Furthermore, all the "measures" imposed on the population are also lies. I support these claims scientifically, mostly by reference to peer reviewed journal articles.
In 2019, WHO scientists reviewed the evidence for utility of all non-pharmaceutical interventions, concluding that they are all without effect.

Given the foregoing, it's no longer possible to view the last two years as well-intentioned errors. Instead, the objectives of the perpetrators are most likely to be totalitarian control over the population by means of mandatory digital ID & cashless, digital currencies (CBDCs).
3. There is no medical or public health emergency. We can & should take back our freedoms with immediate effect. Testing healthy people stops. If you're sick, please stay home. Masks belong in the trash. The covid19 gene-based injections are not recommended & must not be coerced or mandated. Crucially, the vaccine passports database must be destroyed. Economic rectitude is recommended.
4. Serious crimes have obviously been committed. The purpose of this document is to demonstrate that all of the key narrative points about the SARS-CoV-2 virus said to cause the disease covid-19 & the measures imposed to control it are incorrect. Given the sources of these points are scientists, doctors and public health officials, they are not simply mistaken. Instead, they have lied in order to mislead. I believe the motivations of those who I call the perpetrators become clear, once it is internalized that the entire event is based on lies. In recent days, news is breaking that antibodies are present in European blood banks from November, 2019. https://threadreaderapp.com/thread/1503112014700285953.html
The implications are momentous.

In the first three months of the COVID event, I started noticing senior scientific & medical advisors on UK television say things I found disturbing. Hard to put my finger on the specifics, but they included remarks like "because this is a new virus, there won't be any immunity in the population", "everyone is vulnerable" and "in view of the very high lethality of the virus, we are exploring how best to protect the population". I had been reading extensively about the apparent spread of SARS-CoV-2 in China and beyond, and had already arrived at a number of important conclusions. Essentially, I was sure that, objectively, we weren't going to experience a major event, based on the Diamond Princess cruise ship, but what was happening was that, in my view, senior people were acting a lot more frightened than seemed appropriate. Note that not a single member of the crew died and only a minority on the ship even got infected, suggesting substantial prior immunity, a steep age-lethality relationship and an infection fatality ratio not much different, if at all, from prior respiratory virus infections.

It was with this heightened interest that I began close examination of all aspects of the alleged pandemic. I suspected something very bad was happening when the Imperial College (Neil Ferguson) modeling paper was released. This claimed that over 500,000 people in UK would die unless severe "measures" were put in place. Ferguson had over-projected all of the last five disease-related emergencies in the UK, and had been responsible for the destruction of the beef herd through modeling the spread of foot & mouth disease. I had been reading around all sorts of "non-pharmaceutical interventions" (NPIs) and what this had taught me was that there was absolutely no experimental literature around any of those being spoken of, except masks, which were clearly ineffective in blocking respiratory virus transmission. The non-experts in main stream media drew on a very limited group of experts and I noticed that none were immunologists.

I had in parallel watched the evolving scene in Sweden & was pleased to note that their chief epidemiologist, Anders Tegnell, seemed to know what he was doing and had dismissed the panic. I knew he'd been the deputy of Johan Gieseke, his predecessor, who was still around in an emeritus role. Gieseke was also reassuringly calm.

The final straw was when, on March 23 2020, the British prime minister initiated the first "lockdown". This was wholly without precedent. I knew Sweden had rejected them as wholly unnecessary and also extremely damaging. From that day forward, the team from the UK strategic advisory group for emergencies (SAGE) put up one or more members every day to appear alongside the prime minister or the health minister.

These press conferences were meandering affairs and it wasn't clear what purpose they had. The questions asked never sought to place things in context, but instead to always explore the outer edges of possible outcomes and then follow up remarks that didn't seem adequately prepared. In retrospect, I think the aim was to make them the only "must watch" thing on TV and with such a large, captive audience, a form of fear-based hypnosis was instigated. We were much later informed by Matias Desmet that this was indeed the aim, and this process is called "mass formation". https://rokfin.com/stream/9705/Foreign-Agents-10--Covid-and-Mass-Hypnosis . This process can become malignant, as have past beliefs in events that were later conceded to have been episodes of societal madness, like the Salem witch trials, satanic abuse of children and other delusions. Some experts believe that modern societies are more and not less susceptible to such mass panics, because of the ubiquity of easily-controlled messaging (properly termed propaganda, since it was completely deliberate & carefully planned). Despite use of cartoons, this film leans heavily on academic research from luminaries such as Le Bon, Freud, Bernays, Milgram, Asch and later studies. https://rumble.com/vl52me-mass-psychosis-how-an-entire-population-becomes-mentally-ill-by-after-skool.html

It's important to be cautious about the purported importance of "mass formation". In a sense, it might be seen as wholly impersonal and something that is thrown at the population and lands more or less effectively on people at random. Worse, it comes with the notion that, if you are susceptible, it cannot be resisted. There is a contrasting school of thought which holds that IT, data & AI are capable of assembling a "digital prison" which is tailored to each individual & shaped over time by choices that we each make. The outcome isn't in any way preordained. However, incentives & deterrents are associated with innumerable decisions we make, such as how to pay for something, whether we sell our data for tiny rewards, whether we consciously decide to open links suggested for us, leave location services running permanently & more.

https://home.solari.com/control-freedom-happen-one-person-at-a-time-with-ulrike-granogger/
https://home.solari.com/deep-state-tactics-101-part-i-with-catherine-austin-fitts/

As soon as lockdown was initiated, the focus turned full force onto mass testing, especially testing people without symptoms. I knew this didn't make any sense, because if a large enough number of people are tested daily, without knowledge of the false positive rate, we would certainly very quickly be panicked into thinking there were lots of people walking around with the virus, unaware they had it and allegedly spreading it to others.

Once lockdown was in place, in addition to testing, the press conferences focused on numbers in hospital, numbers on ventilators and ultimately the daily deaths "with COVID". Early treatments and improved lifestyle were never spoken of. The first lockdown lasted 12 weeks, with most office staff told to 'work from home' while being paid 'furlough' (a word never before used in Britain). The "fear porn" continued all the way into high summer, long after daily COVID deaths had reached approximately zero, and the introduction of mandatory masking in all public areas in the heat of summer, when they had never been required before, was the last straw for me. It was all theatre and I set out to investigate a couple of core concepts: the "PCR test" and "asymptomatic transmission". I'm embarrassed to say it wasn't until the autumn of 2020 that I had clear in my mind, with mounting horror, that the entire event, if not completely manufactured, as being grossly exaggerated, with the intent of deceiving the entire "liberal democratic West". Scores of countries were economically being squeezed to death. I knew that from a financial perspective, borrowing or printing enough money to subsidize tens of millions to remain as home could not be long sustained without destroying the sovereign currency. Strangely, exchange rates didn't move much, another clue that powerful forces were managing this event as well as its consequences. Around this time, country leaders started talking about "Build Back Better" and Klaus Schwab's Great Reset book appeared.

Around this time, I developed the idea of "The COVID lies". It seemed to me that everything we had been told about the virus wasn't true and also that all the NPIs imposed upon us couldn't work and so were for nothing more than show. As above, repetition and fear were key to instigating "mass formation" as described in detail by Belgian Professor Matias Desmet (https://rokfin.com/stream/9705/Foreign-Agents-10--Covid-and-Mass-Hypnosis). This narrowing of focus, according to Desmet, means those "in the mass" (crowd) are literally incapable of hearing anything which challenges the narrative of which they're convinced. Any explanation other than the truth is marshalled in dismissing rational counter-arguments. Anyone challenging the dominant narrative was attacked, smeared, censored and cancelled on social media and no reasonable and independent voices were ever seen or heard on TV and radio. The conditions required for mass formation to be successful are argued to be high levels of free-floating anxiety, a strong degree of social isolation where devices replace real human interactions and finally, low levels of sense-making, that is, many things do not make sense to many people. When a crisis is dropped into such a population & repeated ad nauseam, it is possible in effect to hypnotize them. Now their anxiety has an obvious focus, which is felt as a relief. The routines- masking, lockdowns, testing, hand sanitizing, etc. - become for some a ritual which provides daily meaning. Finally, so many people are acting the same way and echoing the same lines that they've heard time and again on TV, radio, newspapers and their devices, they begin to feel part of a national effort in a way they've not felt before. This combination, coupled with visible and strong punishment for anyone who questions the narrative or simply refuses to comply, reinforces the group-think. It is, according to the experts, near-impossible to extract this deeply "in the mass". However, there is always a group who never fall for such tricks. Outwardly pleasant and easy-going, they are typically skeptical and go along with things only if they make sense personally, not because an authority figure tells them to. The group in the middle often senses something is wrong, but lacks the courage of their own convictions and tends to side with whatever they're told to do, rather passively. They are not hypnotized, but to third parties, they can seem to be so. Crowd psychology experts encourage those who've seen through the lies to speak out & continue to do so. First, this legitimizes speaking out by all others not persuaded by the narrative and might extract some of the middle group. Even those "in the mass" will be prevented from sinking yet more deeply into the mass, from where those orchestrating events can otherwise prompt such people to commit atrocities.

In the second half of the year, the conversation turned to the oncoming vaccines. Having spent 32 years in pharmaceutical R&D, I knew what we were being told was just lies. It's not possible to bypass a dozen years of careful work or to compress it into a few months. The product that was to emerge was almost certain, to my mind, to be very dangerous. I read my way into this area, and grew more concerned still.

In what follows, I ONLY isolate the major narrative points themselves and show that none of them are true. There was not just a little lying here and there. No, the entire construct was false. I will describe all the main ones. After that, I'll show how the organizers were able to get away with it.

At the conclusion, I believe the reader will share my view that the whole event is manufactured or exaggerated from a mild situation. No alternative views were permitted in the 'public square'. A group of powerful media organizations assembled in 2019 and founded the Trusted News Initiative. The purpose was both to control the mass media message and crush alternative voices from any direction. https://dailyexpose.uk/2021/08/29/the-trusted-news-initiative-a-bbc-led-organisation-censoring-public-health-experts-who-oppose-the-official-narrative-on-covid-19/

All of it was lies. Not mistakes. Many politicians repeated others' lines and might offer as defence that they relied on experts to inform them. Rachel Walensky recently did just that - said that the CDC made vaccination recommendations because CNN published Pfizer's press release saying that their c19 vaccine was 95% effective. You can't make this up. However, those true subject matter experts, such as Dr. Fauci, Sir Patrick Vallance etc. who promoted them from the public health departments knew they were untrue. What possible motive might there have been to create this state of fear? Who must have been involved to have granted authorization to do it?

The question of motive has to arise. I have tried to find benign explanations & failed to do so. The conclusions I'm drawn to logically make very disturbing reading. I look forward to discussing this with Dr. Sheftall and indeed anyone. It's unlikely I am correct on every point. What I am sure of is that the overall picture is one of extreme deception and a highly-organized fraud. I am not alone in reaching this view. This author steps through what they would do in order to take over the world through a simultaneous "coup d'etat" of the liberal democracies. https://boriquagato.substack.com/p/if-i-were-going-to-conquer-you
Robert F Kennedy Jr also summarizes a plausible explanation. https://www.bitchute.com/video/wyFtd4mshFO8/

I appear to be the ONLY former executive-level scientist from big pharma anywhere in the world speaking out. I've invested 2y pro bono in identifying the key elements of the fraud, in the sincere hope I can connect with Dr. Sheftall and other upright individuals who can help bring this to wider attention and ultimately, to a halt and to justice. I can describe a global fraud operating for two years at tremendous cost in lives, the economy and the very structure of human societies can only be undertaken by powerful people, organized for a purpose which is not to the benefit of ordinary people.

Ps: though not all central, there is a large number of ancillary points and I have assembled a few here:

1.   In a series of short films, you will find another team's interpretation of the same fraud, with remarkable similarities. Note in particular, film 2 (3.5min) on non-pharmaceutical interventions: https://www.canadiancovidcarealliance.org/media-resources/pandemic-alternative/

2.   German investigative journalist, Paul Schreyer, shows that this fraud was rehearsed for many years, increasingly with all the stakeholders now running the alleged covid19 fraud: https://wissen-ist-relevant.de/vortrage/paul-schreyer-pandemic-simulation-games-preparation-for-a-new-era/

3.   Why were autopsies strongly discouraged worldwide in 2020 & still today? To cover up the lack of COVID-19 deaths. After vaccination, a large fraction of deaths have been judged to be due to the vaccines & lack of autopsies covers them up, too. https://doctors4covidethics.org/on-covid-vaccines-why-they-cannot-work-and-irrefutable-evidence-of-their-causative-role-in-deaths-after-vaccination/

4. On what basis were "cases" determined purely by the result of one test, much disputed as to its appropriateness? The Nobel Prize winning inventor of the test, Dr. Kary Mullis, stated definitively that the PCR must not be used to diagnose viral illnesses. https://www.youtube.com/watch?v=rXm9kAhNj-4

5. A death from any cause, within 28 days of a positive test for SARS-CoV-2, is recorded as a "COVID death". It's absurd and we have never assigned cause of death like this before, ever. The effect of untrustworthy PCR tests and the arbitrary assignment of a dubious positive as somehow causative of death has been a very effective way to fool and frighten people. Most do not know that there are literally scores of viruses that can infect human airways, some of which in the elderly and infirmed, can give rise to severe illnesses. Even common cold viruses can do this.

6. Hospital treatment protocols, where I have explored them, look designed to kill. In UK, the pathway starts with everyone being tested with untrustworthy PCR tests and these are applied repeatedly for an in-patient. Given 2% of admissions end in a hospital death, repeated poor testing guarantees a lot of "COVID deaths". A patient "diagnosed" as positive for COVID is placed in isolation and visitors are not allowed until they are moribund. A standard treatment involves intravenous midazolam and morphine from a syringe driver, at doses up to 10 x greater than advisable for a patient capable of breathing unaided. This often results in respiratory failure and either immediate death or mechanical ventilation, accompanied by withdrawal of all care, and of course they then expire. It's murder.

Again, in the UK, we have documentary evidence that the UK NHS stockpiled a year's supply of midazolam, by ordering it normally, but banning 2019 prescriptions. In no more than two months in 2020, the entire supply was exhausted by April, and another year's supply was bulk purchased from a generics company in France, cleaning out their stock. Something similar occurred in US hospitals, with ramped cash bonuses for each stage passed, up to & including mechanical ventilation. Mechanical ventilation is rarely appropriate, because covid19 is NOT an obstructive lung disorder. Blood oxygen desaturation is best addressed using non-invasive masks with elevated oxygen levels. We tried this in Italy in Feb 2020 and they then ceased mechanical ventilation within a week, so stark were the differences in outcomes (most ventilated patients died, most masked patients survived). Apparently, the method of treatment they'd been given from "colleagues in Wuhan" was what they called "the Wuhan protocol". In this, the guidance was that the sooner they sedated & ventilated an agitated patient, the better their chances. This was a lie. Panicked patients needed anxiolytics and an oxygen mask, but they were instead killed.

7. I have been incensed by the mis-use of novel, experimental "vaccines" in recovered individuals (they are immune & risks of adverse events are greatly increased, because the body is already poised to attack any cells expressing spike protein). They are also used in pregnant women, who are not at greatly elevated risks from COVID-19, because they tend to be young and healthy. We've NEVER approved the use of experimental agents in pregnant women since thalidomide (1956-62), certainly not without "reproductive toxicology". None of the vaccines have a completed "reprotox package". I filed a short, expert opinion to court with AFLDS on this topic. They also didn't complete an ADME-Tox package. The FOIAed documents obtained in March 2022 show that Pfizer was "planning to study" vaccination in maternity as of April 30 2021. That's after they have manufactured and shipped close to 100 million doses. Finally, the mis-use of these agents in healthy children without question has reverse risk/benefit: they kill far more than the virus could. The whole thing stinks of a purpose different from public health, because if it was a legitimate public health effort, we definitely would NOT do any of these things. Officials lied on the national broadcaster, such as the BBC, smearing people like me, who had written the world's first treatise, explaining some of our concerns. Note that this petition was co-authored by Dr Wolfgang Wodarg, the public health doctor & minor politician from Germany who stopped the fraudulent "swine flu pandemic" in 2009. https://dryburgh.com/mike-yeadon-coronavirus-vaccine-safety-concerns-petition/

8.	Next, two strange occurrences. First, the WHO altered the definition of "immunity", to exclude "natural immunity". (https://peterlegyel.wordpress.com/2021/01/15/who-changes-definition-of-herd-immunity/). That meant that only vaccination could accomplish the goal. They eventually changed this back, but for many, the damage was done and non-experts didn't trust natural immunity, even though it is superior to that from vaccination, because the body has been exposed to all parts of the virus and will therefore respond to any part of it if reinfected. Next, the WHO changed the definition of "pandemic", which previously meant the simultaneously spreading across many countries of a pathogen, causing many cases and deaths. It was changed to eliminate the need for many deaths (see 45min 50 sec Dr Wolfgang Wodarg, interviewed on UK TV in 2010 after the exaggerated swine flu pandemic, which I now believe was something of a rehearsal for the 2020 covid19 pandemic): https://www.expandingawarenessrelations.com/tag/wolfgang/).

This is a critical point, because PCR can be designed against any pathogen and protocols adopted such that a large number of false positives appear. This grants bad actors the ability relatively easily to create the illusion of a pandemic, almost to order. Interestingly, Dr Wodarg recaps his 2009 experiences and shows similarities with recent events in an interview here: https://www.pandata.org/wolfgang-wodarg/

Many people simply don't believe experts when they talk of "very high fraction of positive test results being false positives". I assure you there have genuinely been a number of events where the entire suspected epidemic was an illusion, and 100% of positives were false positives. Here is an example which, when I first read it, get me a crawling sensation. I wonder if it was this genuine event that birthed the method for exaggerating (or even fully faking) a pandemic in which are currently living? https://silview.media/2020/12/26/nyt-2007-faith-in-quick-test-leads-to-epidemic-that-wasnt/   Its also important to note that WHO changed definitions of immunity from "that obtained after natural infection or vaccination" to only mention vaccination. The definition of a vaccine was also changed, so that it wasn't necessary to prevent infection or transmission, whereas traditional vaccines almost always do this. They do so because they prevent the development of clinical illness and, in the case of respiratory viruses at least, lack of symptoms renders the person all but incapable of infecting anyone else.

9.	I noticed early on that Gates said "we won't return to normal until pretty much the whole planet has been vaccinated". This is a bizarre statement from a person with no medical or scientific training (or indeed a college degree in anything). It is never necessary to vaccinate the entire population, when only the elderly and infirm are at serious risk of death if infected. Note that the median age of deaths from / with covid was the same or even older than the median age of death due to all causes. Blair insisted that vaccine passports would be essential to confidence. Again, absurd, especially once we learned that these vaccines do not prevent transmission. Once this became clear, the case for coerced vaccination vanished and this is the present position. Yet, my unvaccinated relatives may not enter the US. The safest person to be around, if you fear infection, isn't a vaccinated person, but a person who is fit and well, with no respiratory symptoms.

10.	The practise of "boosting", giving people dose after dose of poorly-designed agent, ostensibly to reinforce their immunity, has no immunological basis. No genuine immunity wanes in a few months, sometimes even a few weeks. The perpetrators have exploited the public's understanding of the annual influenza vaccine and somehow normalised something that is dangerous and ineffective. I also noticed that early on, in discussing immunity, antibodies were the discussion topic. T-cells were an "extremist plot". This is another absurdity. I can assemble expert witnesses who will attest alongside me that blood-based antibodies are relatively unimportant, potentially irrelevant to infection by respiratory viruses. This is because the virus infects the air side of the airways and blood-based antibodies cannot leave the blood and enter this "compartment". Blood antibodies and respiratory viruses never meet except under unusual circumstances. On the contrary, T-cells leave the blood and migrate through infected airway tissue, removing infected cells.

11.　　Prof Neil Ferguson (Imperial) has a poor record of modelling & predictions: https://covid19up.org/neil-ferguson-fear-driven-predictions/

12.　　Frighteningly prescient testimony from a former WHO staffer, Jane Burgermeister, in 2010. Her understanding was that respiratory virus pandemics will be used to force near universal vaccination and that this had sinister motives. https://brandnewtube.com/watch/jane-bu-rgermeister-forced-vax-warning-february-15-2010_Con7FXMOCvgW8Or.html I dismissed this the first time I saw it. Many of us turn away instinctively from evil because we cannot or do not want to believe that other humans are capable of that which our logic tells us is happening. I now no longer reject it. It fits far too well with the totally independent Paul Schreyer documentary.

13.　　Another doctor made similar claims, Dr Rima Laibow. This testimony speaks of population rejection, and like Jane Burgermeister, locates the fraud in a conceptual world government. Again, one can reject it, or consider it alongside other pieces of information. https://www.brandnewtube.com/watch/jesse-ventura-meets-dr-rima-laibow_kL2AlR=

14.　　I think it's worth developing this theme of turning away from evidence of sheer evil. I have to say more, because it is THE pressing issue today. The evidence I set forth makes it perfectly plain that the entire world is being lied to in ways that led predictably to huge suffering and death. Given none of the "measures" imposed could have mitigated illness and death from a respiratory virus, the only outcome was to be fracturing of civil society and damage, potentially fatal, to the economy and financial system. I emphasise again here that WHO scientists had conducted a detailed review of control measures for respiratory virus epidemics and pandemics as recently as 2019 and that concluded that no imposed measures make any difference at all. The claims made for control in Wuhan are not credible. The stakeholders who must have approved this action own or control the majority of the world's capital and assets. Their motivation cannot be for money, for they stand astride the money-creating apparatus in the central and private banks. Equally, it cannot be to obtain gross control over the population, since they already demonstrably have that. This is what leads me inexorably to propose that the motives behind this are terrible. At very least, to secure totalitarian control through mandatory, digital ID (in the guise of useless vaccine passports, useless because none of these so-called vaccines reduce transmission, the only possibly justification for them). Add to this a "financial great reset" with withdrawal of cash and introduction of central bank digital currencies and we have a wholly controlled population, controlled automatically without human intervention on the ground. All that's needed is to require the population to show their health passport or else they will not be allowed to cross a regulated threshold, like accessing a food store, or make a transaction using digital money, unless the AI algorithm permits it. If those operating this takeover of humanity wished then to eliminate a portion of the population, with plausible deniability, I doubt a more propitious starting point could be had. I do not believe it's a fault in those who fall for the narrative that they cannot see the lies. People want to believe that governments and experts, for all their well-known flaws and occasionally uncovered corruption, are trying to do the best they can and cannot accept the truth, that there is a group of powerful people who regard the ordinary members of the public as surplus to requirements. They want to deny evil, because it makes them feel bad, sad, uncomfortable to think about the world this way. They want to deny reality and that's their coping mechanism which is being exploited by the perpetrators of evil. It gives cloak of invisibility to those who want to commit mass murder, quite literally, since so many people are so willing to imagine that it is not happening.

15.　　It is not clear to me what to do with the information I've gathered here. I believe that a calm review of the summary, which I call "The COVID lies" will result in any open-minded person agreeing that we all have been subjected to a monstrous fraud, with lethal consequences and that there is overwhelming evidence of long-term planning and deliberately injurious acts. There is no easy way to say that, but it could be represented objectively & taught, in the manner of a workshop, so that participants get to derive their own conclusions (albeit being led by the evidence). I doubt just talking to a group of people who hold the narrative view as "true" would respond at all well to this, delivered as a lecture. Nobody wants to accept they've been fooled, even if the blow is softened by telling them that this has been brought about by highly experienced professionals in the covert services & has required huge amounts of money to buy off several groups. But ignoring this and hoping it will go away is naïve and very dangerous for us all. The perpetrators have not gone away and will likely return in the fall. I expect this year or the next will see them assume totalitarian tyranny, if we have not, before then, "inoculated" important stakeholder groups to understand whats happened so far and to be alert to the many potential presentation of the next fear-provoking episode. On the positive side, an increasing number of people have detected that fraud is ongoing. This is a particularly good example, from the financial analysts community, which refers to life insurance claims among many other pieces of evidence of wrong-doing: https://rumble.com/vwjmjm-bombshell-naomi-wolf-interviews-edward-dowd-about-pfizer-fraud-and-criminal.html

Chapter 2

13 COVID Lies   -Dr. Michael Yeadon

1. SARS-CoV-2 has such a high lethality that every measure must be taken to save lives.

It was essential to claim high lethality in order that unprecedented responses may seem justified.

To "pep up" the claim, recall "falling man" in Wuhan? The person was allegedly sick but walking about, before falling dead on their face. That was never real.

Note, COVID-19 is the disease resulting from infection with the virus, SARS-CoV-2. They are often used interchangeably. Sometimes it doesn't matter but the confusion was sewn deliberately.

Early estimates of lethality were very high, in some reports, an "infection fatality rate" of 3%. Seasonal influenza is generally considered to have a typical IFR of 0.1%. That means some seasons, IFR for 'flu may be 0.3% and other times, 0.05% or lower.

In practice, and this was usual, estimates of IFR for COVID-19 (Wuhan strain) were revised downwards repeatedly and now are generally recognized as in the range 0.1-0.3%. It cannot now be argued that it is significantly different from some seasonal influenza epidemics. Why then have we all but destroyed the modern world over it?

Dr. Sheftall adds: While living in Phnom Penh, Cambodia, the news of the outbreak on the Princess Cruise Lines and its subsequent quarantine in Yokohama was updated every day. Having great suspicions about the infection fatality rates being advanced by the typical authorities such as the China Medical Authority (at 4%), I got to work calculating my own IFR. In short, I learned very soon that the authorities were engaged in selection bias due to not counting the asymptomatic "infected" or they were deliberately trying to instill fear in the population. I favored the former at first but later realized it was a deliberate effort to control large populations. From the good work done by crews of Japanese medical personnel boarding the ship every day and testing as many passengers and crew as they could, I got the information on number infected (and, crucially, number not infected) and number died and calculated the IFR to be .1% with a few justifiable assumptions and a little bit of common sense. I shared my findings on March 8, 2020. Dr. Michael Levitt calculated the IFR from the same cruise ship data (with slightly different assumptions) and arrived at an IFR of .2%. Dr. Ioannidis wrote an article in STAT News in which he argued the IFR to be.

These other two very accomplished gentlemen- Dr. Levitt shared the 19 Nobel Prize in Chemistry and Dr. Ioannidis is a legend in epidemiological circles- would agree that this was very simple stuff, requiring nothing more than simple arithmetic, but of great importance. The implications of getting the IFR significantly wrong in either direction would be dire as it relates to the policies instituted to combat the looming pandemic. Dr. Yeadon continues: The perpetrators knew that lethality estimates of new respiratory viral illnesses ALWAYS start high and reduce. This is because, early on, we do not have any estimate of the number of people infected but not seriously ill & the number infected with no symptoms at all.

They created the impression of extreme danger, which was never true. This is such a crucial point, for once one sees it for what it is, the rest of the narrative is superfluous.

Dr John Ioannidis is one of the world's most-published epidemiologists and he has been scathing about the inappropriate responses to a novel virus of not particularly unusual lethality. Like most respiratory viruses, SARS-CoV-2 represents no serious health threat to those under 60y, certainly not children, and is a serious threat only to those nearing the end of their lives by virtue of age and multiple comorbidities. https://www.sciencedirect.com/science/article/pii/S0013935120307854

Dr Ioannidis current estimate of global infection fatality rate is around 0.15%. For reference, a typical seasonal influenza outbreak has a typical IFR of around 0.1%, but can be markedly worse in bad winters. https://onlinelibrary.wiley.com/doi/10.1111/eci.13554

2. Because this is a new virus, there will be no prior immunity in the population.
Seems reasonable, doesn't it? This remark, made repeatedly early on, aimed to squash any notion that there was a degree of "prior immunity" in the population.

Prior immunity and natural immunity are only now, two years in, not considered "misinformation".

Within a few months, multiple publications showed that a large minority (ranging 30-50%, some later said even more) of the population had T-cells in their blood which recognized various pieces of the viral protein (synthesized, as no one seemed to have any real virus isolates to use).

While some people argued that recognition by T-cells didn't mean functional immunity, really it does.

We were prevented from learning that we already knew of six coronaviruses, four of which cause "common colds", which in the elderly & infirmed can cause death.

Dr. Sheftall adds: A revealing graphic arose out of one of the studies to which Dr. Yeadon is referring. It is from a very important paper by Sette, Crotty et al (Sette, 2020).

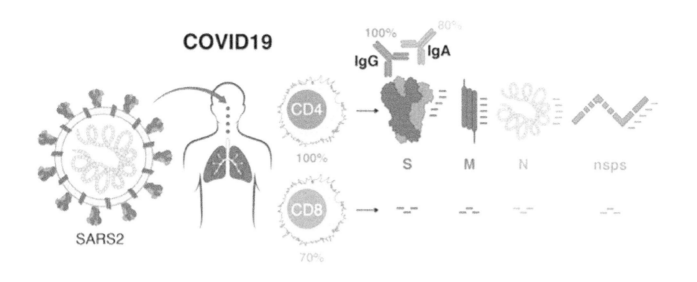

I used this schematic over and over again in my videos and live presentations from the date it appeared in the paper referenced above. Its implications and applications are many. I referred to this and one other related slide as "the two most important slides of the pandemic" early on and in my discussions with Dr. Bhattacharya later in the pandemic. I believe this ranking is justified because the two reveal so much truth about the human immunological response while exposing so much malfeasance and collusion by those pushing the false narrative Dr. Yeadon so bravely and insightfully warned us about very early on. The sister slide to this one shows 23 patients who were still alive 17 years after recovering from SARS-1 who are still protected against SARS-1, but also protected against SARS-2 without having ever been exposed to it due to the similarity of the N protein that is almost identical in the two viruses.

The schematic above spells out how this happens. It shows the differences and similarities between study participants who had been exposed to the SARS-2 virus, pictured on top, and those who had not been exposed, on the bottom.

The top shows what we would expect. In 100% and 80% of the exposed participants, a hearty IgG and IgA response to the spike protein was measured in blood samples. Also, a strong (5 hash marks) CD4 (the T-helper subgroup) response was shown toward the S (spike), the 'M' (radius of curvature), the 'N' (RNA stabilizing), and the nonstructural proteins in 100% of the participants. In 70%, a 3 hash CD8 (T-killer) subset presence was found to all of these proteins. As I said, all of this is entirely expected upon exposure to the virus. It's the bottom half that turns this slide into the most important of the pandemic. It refutes almost everything the evil people did to distort the science.

It shows a 3 or 4 hash mark CD4 presence toward the S, M and NSPs OF SARS-2! in 50% of those participants who had never been exposed to the SARS-2 virus. And 20% had CD8 presence for these proteins.

How could that be if none of these participants had ever been exposed to SARS-2? It's really very simple. Because SARS-2 is a member of a family of viruses known as the Coronaviridae, it shares characteristics with other members of that family (such as those that cause the common cold with which many participants had battled earlier in their lives) in the same way that people from the same human family usually resemble each other due to homology in their genotypes, being from the same parents.

So when people started referring to SARS-2 as a "novel coronavirus", my antenna went up and I know Dr. Yeadon's did too. The term is nonsensical. If it's a coronavirus it's going to have a lot in common with other coronaviruses or it wouldn't be a coronavirus. That's how scientists put these things in families and subgroups together; based on their genetic commonality which itself determines their morphological similarity.

They were trying to make it out like this virus was new to the degree that made it dangerous because new is potentially dangerous when you're talking about viruses. WHO Director Tedros even said, "COVID-19 is a new virus and nobody has immunity to it" which was completely wrong, of course. In fact, the opposite was true. A significant number of people, on the order of 1/3 of the population of different countries around the world, was protected before the virus appeared on their shores. Those people had mounted a protective T cell response to proteins which were identical or similar enough to analogous proteins in the SARS-2 virus. I'm talking about being protected against a virus before it came into existence! So the claim by the evildoers that there was no prior protection, was always a lie that made no sense. The viruses we encounter are offspring from common ancestors who gave rise to cousins we have had to fend off in our past, cousins that are made up of proteins like the N protein of SARS-1 and SARS-2 that have not changed over many years. It would go against immunological principles to think no one in a large population had at least some prior cross protection. How many? Look at the schematic above. Half of the unexposed participants had T helper cells directed against the proteins of SARS-2and 20% had T killers. There were no circulating antibodies, of course but that doesn't matter.

Because the proteins in the original virus elicited clonal expansion and memory in the person infected, when that same person gets infected with a related virus using the same protein or one very similar, that person is protected against both the original virus and the new virus through something come to be known as cross-reactivity. The analogy that's always used is that of a lock and key. The virus protein is the lock and the body makes lots of keys to it so that the keys can rapidly open it the next time it invades the body. If another very similar lock comes calling, the keys made for the original might open that lock too and destroy it, in which case the person would be protected against the second intruder.

The lock and key analogy is ok for our purposes but it's terribly oversimplified. The surfaces of proteins are composed of complex electron probability clouds whose interactions with the clouds surrounding antigen binding domains of antibodies and T cell receptors is only partially-understood. There's lots quantum mechanics going on here and we have only a vague understanding of the interaction based on probabilities.

Nevertheless, it is easy to show that large fractions of populations were never at risk of getting COVID-19 and should never been forced to get the vaccine at the threat of losing their freedoms and other civil liberties and their means of making a living. If you'll pardon me, Dr. Fauci, Dr. Birx, all of the TV doctors (the M.D.T.V. Mafia), and all the others you will learn about shortly, who pushed for universal vaccination despite knowing about the phenomenon of cross reactivity protection and the protection one acquires from exposure to the actual virus, those people deserve to be punished very severely; prison for life if they pushed these unnecessary vaccines, knowing there were hundreds of millions of people just in the U.S. who were already protected and incapable of spreading the virus to others and who did not need to receive the vaccine. And you want to know something? They ALL knew this freshman level stuff and should be put behind the walls for the remainder of their natural lives. If you think I'm being hyperbolic, think again. What these people did while knowing better, resulted in the deaths of hundreds of thousands of people and counting and that's just from the vaccines. When we talk about the lockdowns, the numbers get into the hundreds of millions and counting.

I coined a term "immunity-in-place" to describe these people when I crunched the numbers for the Diamond Princess Cruise ship and later in March when it was the only possible reason why some residents of the Washington State nursing homes were not getting infected with the virus when others across the hall were getting infected and dying from it. Their having immunity-in-place was the only explanation for why people on the cruise ship who were packed in like sardines with the sick ones and nursing home residents breathing in millions of viruses every minute of the day were not testing positive, getting sick, and dying. And then you've got Dr. Fauci coming on TV every day saying everyone has to get vaccinated even if they got the disease and recovered, let alone if they had immunity-in-place (which he never recognized). The amount of evil associated with this was something I grappled with from the beginning and still do. We must do something about this in the way of not letting the SARS-2 marauders get away with this- something akin to the Nuremburg Trials- so people think twice before they ever think of doing this again.

3. This virus does not discriminate. No one is at safe until everyone is safe.

This claim was always absurd. The lethality of this virus, as is common with respiratory viruses, is at least 1000X less in young, healthy people than in elderly people with multiple comorbidities.

In short, almost no one who wasn't close to the end of their lives were at risk of severe outcomes & death. In middle-aged individuals, obesity is a risk factor, as it is for a handful of other causes of death.

This intriguing review details how the initial modeling induced fear and provided the excuse for heavy-handed measures especially "lockdown". It was however just that: an excuse. All experienced public health experts knew that lockdown was absurd, ineffective and hugely destructive. There's no way to sugar-coat this. It was wrong before it was ordered and it's necessary to examine why those who knew did not protest. It's almost as if they were complicit.

4. People can carry this virus with no signs and infect others: asymptomatic transmission.

This is the central conceptual deceit. If true, then anyone might infect & kill you.

Falsely claimed asymptomatic transmission underscores almost every intrusion: masking, mass testing, lockdowns, border restrictions, school closures, even vaccine passports.

The best evidence comes from a meta-analysis of a larger number of good studies, examining how often a person testing positive went on to infect a family member (they compared as potential sources of infection people who had symptoms with those who did not have symptoms). ONLY those WITH symptoms were able to infect a family member at any rate that mattered.

Asymptomatic transmission is epidemiologically irrelevant. It's not necessary to argue it never happens, it's enough to show that if it occurs at all, it is so rare as to not be worth measuring.

In this case, we also have Fauci and a WHO doctor telling us exactly this. Also, I show why it is like it is. It's very clear.

Dr. Sheftall adds: I have a slight disagreement with Dr. Yeadon here. First of all, in principle, Dr. Yeadon is correct. I was on his side until very recently. In my video discussions with Dr. Jay Bhattacharya that have taken place throughout 2022 and total 24 hours at this point, I argued that it would be a first principles violation for a virus such as SARS-2 to transmit asymptomatically. The reason for this is that it takes more of a viral load to transmit than it does to cause symptoms. Jay had some evidence that there *was* some asymptomatic transmission, however. We fought and fought over this. Note: Fighting with Jay is full of smiles. The meanest thing we say to each other is, "are you sure?" He is such a fine gentleman.

We never resolved this disagreement. I would come up with a thought experiment that seemed fail-safe but Jay had the data. I think I have the answer now, and I have to credit another fine gentleman, Steven Quay, M.D., PhD, for leading me to it.

Both Jay and I were right. There *is* some asymptomatic transmission- more than a little- and I was right that it *would* be a first principles violation, if it was not for a little segment of the SARS-2 genome called orf-8. (orf stands for "open reading frame") It's a little piece that inhibits us from feeling symptoms mediated by interferons. Here's a picture of it:

The picture is not that important but the fact that orf-8 is present there is very important. Making a virus that can transmit asymptomatically is one of the two gain of function that are universally frowned upon/illegal because it is essential to the construction of bioweapons. With bioweapons, you want a virus that can spread without your opponents knowing whom to avoid. It's a real no-no.

Two graduate student papers were written in Chinese without being translated that talked about enhancing orf-8–like capability at the Wuhan lab. Dr. Quay had them translated and we talked about it in a recent discussion we had (note: my conversations with Drs. Bhattacharya and Quay can be found at DrReidSheftall.substack.com).

I looked through the literature and I couldn't find another respiratory virus similar to SARS-2 where the asymptomatic were able to transmit the virus. So Dr. Yeadon, Dr. Bhattacharya and myself are all right. This is a good lesson in sticking to your guns and not accepting something that violates first principles

5. The PCR test selectively identifies people with clinical infections.

This is the central operational deceit.

If true, we could detect risky people & isolate them. We could diagnose accurately and also count the number of deaths.

Polymerase chain reaction, at its best, can confirm the presence of genetic information in a clean sample & is useful in forensics for that reason. It involves cycle after cycle of amplification, copying the starting material at the beginning of each cycle.

The inventor of the PCR test, Kary Mullis, won a Nobel Prize for it and often criticised Fauci for mis-using that test to diagnose AIDS patients, which Mullis insisted was inappropriate.

In a 'dirty' clinical sample, however, there is more than a possible piece of, or a whole, virus which might replicate. There are bacteria, fungi, other viruses, human cells, mucus and more. It's not possible unequivocally to know, if a test is judged "positive" after many cycles, what it was that was amplified to give the signal at the end that we call positive.

In mass testing mode, commonly used, no one ever runs so-called "positive controls" through the chain of custody. That's diagnostic testing 101. It's a deception.

Every test has an "operational false positive rate" (oFPR), where some unknown % of samples turn positive, even if there is no virus present. A good oFPR would be less than 1%, but is it 0.8% or 0.1%? If you test 100,000 samples daily, and the oFPR is 0.8%, you will get 800 positive tests or "cases", even if there is no virus in the entire community. Often, the "positivity", the fraction of tests that are positive, is in that range, sub-1% or low single digit %. I believe much or all of that can be caused by false positives. Note, criminals can manipulate the content of the test kits because there are very few providers in a territory, often just one. The conditions for running the test are also subject to variation by the authorities, like the CDC.

You can be genuinely positive, yet not ill. There is no lower limit of true detection below which you'd be declared to have some copies of the virus, but declared clinically well. It's an absurd idea.

You can have no virus yet test positive (with or without symptoms). All of these are swept together and called "confirmed covid19 cases". If you die in the next 28days, you're said to be a "covid death", no matter what the cause.

Those using the test kits provided commercially are what are called "black box". They are unable to say what is in the kit, because this is proprietary. The original "methods paper" was published in 48h, making a mockery of claimed peer review, by a Berlin lab headed by Prof Christian Drosten, scientific advisor to Angela Merkel of Germany.

The paper was comprehensively rebutted by an international team https://cormandrostenreview.com/

The WHO released a series of guidance notes on PCR, and it was clear that their technical staff did not approve of mass testing the population, because it's possible to return wholly false positives. Indeed, at times of low genuine prevalence, that's all they can be.

https://apps.who.int/iris/bitstream/handle/10665/334254/WHO-2019-nCoV-laboratory-2020.6-eng.pdf?sequence=1&isAllowed=y

I often wonder if this real-life example of a PCR-based testing system which returned 100% false positives, yet convinced a major hospital that they had a huge disease outbreak for weeks might have been the inspiration for the untrustworthy methods used in the covid-19 deception?

https://eumeswill.wordpress.com/2020/08/11/faith-in-quick-test-leads-to-epidemic-that-wasnt/

Drosten also led the TV publicity around the idea of asymptomatic transmission. One lucky scientist is at the centre of the two most important deceptions in the entire covid19 event!

Professor Norman Fenton here presents a multi-part lecture with two main elements. First, he describes how mass testing of people with no symptoms unavoidably drives up the proportion of positive PCR test results which are false.

https://rumble.com/vtxi1h-open-science-sessions-how-flawed-data-has-driven-the-narrative.html

The second part deals with the possibility that data fraud entirely accounts for the apparent efficacy of the vaccines, while attempting to hide vaccine deaths, by classifying them as unvaccinated for 14 days after injection.

6. Masks are effective in preventing the spread of this virus.

This is mostly used to maintain the illusion of danger. You see other people wearing masks & feel afraid. Complying is also a measure of whether you do what you're told, especially if the measure is useless.

We have known for decades that surgical masks worn in medical theatres do not stop respiratory virus transmission. Masks were tested across a series of operations by doctors at the Royal College of Surgeons (UK). No difference in post-operative infection rate was seen by mask use.

Cloth masks definitely don't stop respiratory virus transmission as shown by several large, randomized trials. If anything, they increase risk of lung infections. The authorities have mostly conceded on cloth masks.

Some people speak of "source control", catching droplets. Problem is, there is no evidence that significant transmission takes place via droplets. . Equally, there is no evidence it occurs via fine aerosols. No one finds it on masks, or on air filters in hospital wards of covid patients, either. Where is the virus?

It's not necessary to use up time on this topic. It was known long before covid19 that face masks don't do anything.

Many don't know that blue medical masks aren't filters. Your inspired and expired air moves in and out between the mask & your face. They are splashguards, that's all.

This is a good review of the findings with masks in respiratory viruses by a recognized expert in the field. No effect.

https://pubmed.ncbi.nlm.nih.gov/33215698/

Neither masks nor lockdowns prevented the spread of the virus. A review and summary of 400 papers:

https://brownstone.org/articles/more-than-400-studies-on-the-failure-of-compulsory-covid-interventions/

Dr. Sheftall adds: I agree that we don't need to waste time on this. I would only add that several meta-analyses randomized controlled trials were performed over the 72 years preceding COVID-19 and none showed any significant reduction in the spread of laboratory-confirmed respiratory viruses (influenza at the time). The testing of masks in the last two years was superfluous. Even with the political zealots cheating on all the trials, they couldn't show any benefit.   Here are the 72 years-wor

- Quotes from the studies I am referring to, looking at RCT (randomized controlled trials) over 72 years of literature. 1., " Although mechanistic studies support the potential effect of hand hygiene or face masks, evidence from 14 randomized controlled trials of these measures did not support a substantial effect on transmission of laboratory-confirmed influenza." 2., "The evidence from RCTs suggested that the use of face masks either by infected persons or by uninfected persons does not have a substantial effect on influenza transmission". 3.,"In our systematic review, we identified 10 RCTs that reported estimates of the effectiveness of face masks in reducing laboratory-confirmed influenza virus infections in the community from literature published during 1946–July 27, 2018. In pooled analysis, we found no significant reduction in influenza transmission with the use of face masks." 4., " The overall reduction in ILI or laboratory-confirmed influenza cases in the face mask group was not significant in either studies (9,10)" From Emerging Infectious Diseases/NIH/U.S. National Library of Medicine
- https://www.ncbi.nlm.nih.gov/pmc/articles/PMC7181938/

All they had to do was check the literature. I put this in a video I made in April, 2020. And, no, the 2022 Bangladesh study didn't show any benefit. It had more holes in it than a BB gun target at 10 feet.

1. **Lockdowns slow down the spread and reduce the number of cases and deaths.**

The most impactful yet wasteful intervention, accomplishing nothing useful.

Useful to the perpetrators, wishing to damage the economy and reduce interpersonal contacts. This measure was surprisingly tolerated in many wealthy countries, because "furlough" schemes were put in place, compensating many people for not working, or requiring them to work from home.

The measure, though among the most repressive acts ever imposed on citizens in a democracy, was intuitively reasonable to many. This is an example of how far off-course uninformed intuition can be.

The core idea was simple. Respiratory viruses are transmitted from person to person. Reducing the average number of contacts surely reduces transmission?

Actually, it doesn't, because the transmission concept is wrong. Transmission is from a SYMPTOMATIC person to a susceptible person. Those with symptoms are UNWELL. They remain at home in most cases with no action from the government. Transmission occurred mostly in institutions where sick people and susceptible people are forced into contact: hospitals, care homes and domestic settings.

A general lockdown had no detectable impact on epidemic spreading, cases, hospitalizations & deaths.

This is now widely accepted, after a meta-analysis by Johns Hopkins University (interestingly, as the JHU repeatedly features as actors in the Paul Schreyer documentary).

https://www.acsh.org/news/2022/02/16/johns-hopkins-lockdown-analysis-16135

This is because those involved in the vast bulk of human-to-human contacts are fit and well and such contacts didn't result in transmission. Essentially, if you're fooled by the "asymptomatic transmission" lie, then lockdown might make sense. However, since it is epidemiologically irrelevant, lockdowns can never work and of course all the voluminous literature confirms this.

This concept is unequivocally known to multiple public health scientists and doctors. This is why "lockdown" has never been tried.

Importantly, the WHO scientists drafted a detailed review of all the non-pharmaceutical interventions (NPIs) in 2019 and distributed copies of the report to all member states.

This means that ALL member states knew, late in 2019, that masks, lockdowns, border restrictions and business or school closures were already known to be futile. Only "stay home of you're sick" works at all, and people don't need to be told this, for they are too unwell to go out.

https://apps.who.int/iris/handle/10665/329439?search-result=true&query=Non+pharmaceutical+interventions+2018&scope=&rpp=10&sort_by=score&order=desc

Dr. Sheftall adds: There's nothing to add here. I think we just experienced the brilliance of Dr. Michael Yeadon- a perfect explanation of why lockdowns made no sense from the beginning, beautiful in its simplicity.

I disagree with the JHU study, however. It is my contention that lockdowns caused more harm than good (the economics professor from Hopkins found a .2% benefit).

Early data proved my suspicions correct. They showed clearly that those who stayed home got the sickest, were hospitalized more often, and succumbed to the illness more often than those who were allowed to move freely about the community. I'm not talking about deaths from suicide or drug overdoses and certainly not from the avalanche of collateral damage the lockdowns caused such as starvation and cancer due to the moratoriums imposed by the same people who gave the lockdown orders. I'm talking about from COVID-19.

Yes, essential employees who were required to continue in their jobs in the community did better than those who were locked down at home. As far as I know, I am the only person making this claim but I don't think I'm going out on a limb in making it. Lockdowns cannot work for the same reason that plexi-glass guards around office desks could not work and were, in fact, the exact opposite of what needed to be done. In a word, they both create stagnant pockets of air when what you want is high ventilation because this will keep the density of viral particles the lowest. Stagnant air accumulates viral particles in the same way that a 20 meter by 20 meter patch of soft sand that runners are forced to run through in a cross country race will have more runners in it than any other 20 x 20 patch of firm grass. Lockdowns force many people into a place with stagnant air and a higher density of virus particles. It's the worst thing you can do. Worse yet, if one of them gets sick, they will exhale virus-laden breath into the poorly-ventilated space. This causes the concentration of virus to increase rapidly with time until it exceeds the threshold necessary for infection to take hold in a vulnerable person. Sure! Why don't we bring Junior home from college with the sniffles where he just caught the virus and lock him down with grandma! Can you think of a stupider idea than that?

On March 17, 2020, I tried to enlighten the world as to the folly of lockdowns by writing two hosts at FOX and two at CNN. I requested just five minutes in their offices to explain that lockdowns would not work and would cause "death and destruction on a biblical scale". None of the four wrote me back. I also wrote to the White House but didn't hear from them either. In retrospect, I should have gotten on a plane in Phnom Penh and flown to New York. I must have waited more than a month for them to write me back until I realized a screener probably put my emails in a reject folder or deleted them. They probably get 5,000 emails a day.

By then, we were in late April, already heavy into the lockdowns which had been renewed after the initial two weeks. I was reduced to writing posts on Facebook and posting videos on YouTube. My first video was 4 hours long and entitled, "Stop the SARS-2 Stupidity, Doctors. You are Killing People!" With a title like that, it didn't stay up long.

Here is the early data that came in, proving my suspicions correct that the lockdowns caused more harm than good, in and of themselves (i.e. not including collateral damage, which dwarfs the relatively small effect, unnoticeable at cursory glance or on any graph of cases vs. time.

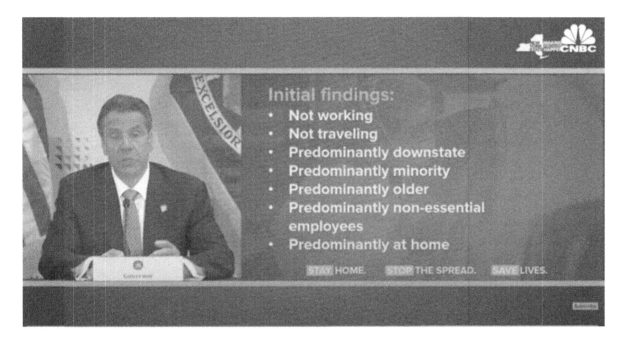

This shows the people who did the worst were not working, predominantly non-essential employees, and predominantly at home. I saw this live on CNBC from Cambodia. It was surreal watching Governor Cuomo try to tell people to "Stay home, Save Lives" (look at the bottom line) while a centimeter above this line it lists the characteristics of the people who were getting hospitalized and dying most often as "Predominantly at home". I was the only person who spoke up about this, as far as I could tell. People were giving these guys a pass on everything they said and did, no matter how idiotic it was or maybe they just didn't notice. Either way, the degree of stupidity associated with this fraud was mind boggling.

8. There are unfortunately no treatments for covid beyond support in hospital.
Reinforced the idea that it was vital to avoid catching the virus.
Legally, it was essential for the perpetrators bringing forward novel vaccines that there be no viable treatments. Had there been even one, the regulatory route of Emergency Use Authorisation would not have been available.

In my opinion, while all these measures were destructive and cruel, active deprivation of access to experimentally applied but otherwise known safe and effective early treatments led directly to millions of avoidable deaths worldwide. In my mind, this is a policy of mass murder.

Contrasting with the official narrative, the therapeutic value of early treatment was already understood and demonstrated empirically during spring 2020. Since then, a sizeable handful of well-understood, off-patent, low-cost and safe oral treatments have been characterised.

The official position was that the disease covid19 could not be treated and the patient only "supported", often by mechanical ventilation. Ventilation is wholly inappropriate because covid19 is rarely an obstructive airway disease, yet has a high associated morbidity and mortality. An oxygen mask is greatly preferred.

In my view, due to the very large amount of empirical treatment and good communication, covid19 is the most treatable respiratory viral illness ever. We knew in the first 3 months of 2020 that hydroxychloroquine, zinc and azithromycin were empirically useful, provided treatment was started early and tackled rationally.

https://pubmed.ncbi.nlm.nih.gov/32771461/

adv

It's very important to note that it has been known for a decade and more that elevating intracellular zinc acts to suppress viral replication. https://journals.plos.org/plospathogens/article?id=10.1371/journal.ppat.1001176

There is no question that senior advisors to a range of governments knew that so-called "zinc ionophores", compounds which open channels to allow certain dissolved minerals to cross cell membranes, were useful in SARS (2003) and should be expected also to be therapeutically useful in SAR-CoV-2 infection.

This is a starting point for all of the clinical trials in covid-19, including especially ivermectin and hydroxychloroquine (which are zinc ionophores).

https://c19early.com/

https://journals.lww.com/americantherapeutics/Fulltext/2021/08000/Ivermectin_for_Prevention_and_Treatment_of.7.aspx

It should be noted that using known safe agents for experimental purposes as a priority has always been an established ethical medical practice & is known as "off label prescribing".

9.   It's not certain if you can get the virus more than once.

The idea of natural immunity was flatly denied and the absurd idea that you might get the same virus twice was established.

Ramped up the fear, which might otherwise pass swiftly.Those with even a basic grasp of mammalian immunology knew that senior advisors to government, speaking in uncertain terms on this question, were lying. Certainly, in the author's case, it was a pivotal point. I share a foundational education in UK universities at the same time as the UK government's Chief Scientific Advisor. This shared education meant we'd have had the same set texts. I reasoned that he knew what I knew and vice versa. I was as sure as it's possible to be that it wouldn't be possible to get clinically unwell twice in response to the same virus, or close-in variants of it. I was right. He was lying.

There have been scores of peer reviewed journal articles on this topic. Very few clinically-important reinfections have ever been confirmed.

https://brownstone.org/articles/how-likely-is-reinfection-following-covid-recovery/

Beating off a respiratory virus infection leaves almost everyone with acquired immunity which is complete, powerful and durable.

You wouldn't know it for the misdirection around antibodies in blood but such antibodies are not considered pivotally important in host immunity. Secreted antibodies in airway surface liquid of the IgA isotype certainly, but most important are memory T-cells.
https://www.medrxiv.org/content/10.1101/2020.11.02.20222778v1

Those infected with SARS in 2003 still had clear evidence of robust, T-cell mediated immunity 17 years later.
https://www.nature.com/articles/s41586-020-2550-z

Dr. Sheftall adds: In a sea of absurd claims, this was one of the most outlandish. As late as September 28, 2020, the M.D.T.V. Mafia, in particular, Drs. Reiner and Haseltine and Dr. Fauci were claiming 90% of the people in the US were still vulnerable and that we were very far away from Herd immunity. They based this claim on serological sampling studies such as the one below by Dr. Julie Parsonnet's team at Stanford. This grossly undercounts those exposed because checking antibodies in the blood doesn't take into account 1) that antibodies only last about 90 days in the serum, 2) B and T cell memory lines (the point being here that even if there are no antibodies in a patient's blood, it doesn't mean he isn't protected by clonal memory), 3) Immunity-in-place. About a third of the US population or 120 million people were protected from this before the virus arrived on our shores as I have explained. Parsonnet's study concluded that only 32.4 million people were protected when the actual number was about 275 million. (155 million exposed + 120 million with immunity-in-place).

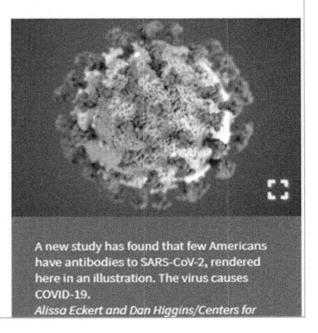

Fewer than 1 in 10 Americans have antibodies to coronavirus, study finds

In a nationally representative analysis of coronavirus antibodies, researchers also found high rates of infection among Black and Hispanic people, and in densely populated areas.

SEP 28 2020

About 9% of people nationwide have been infected with the coronavirus, according to a new study led by Stanford School of Medicine investigators.

"This is the largest study to date to confirm that we are nowhere near herd immunity," said Julie Parsonnet, MD, professor of medicine and of epidemiology and population health, referring to the point at which a large part of the population becomes immune to a specific disease. Scientists estimate that 60%-70% of the population must have antibodies to the coronavirus before COVID-19, the disease the virus causes, fades, said Parsonnet, a co-author of the study.

A new study has found that few Americans have antibodies to SARS-CoV-2, rendered here in an illustration. The virus causes COVID-19.
Alissa Eckert and Dan Higgins/Centers for

173

I made a few videos about this because it was so important for a few major reasons. One was that we were, in fact very close to herd immunity and reached it only a few months later on January 11, 2021, only nine months after the initial outbreak (sometimes called the "first wave" (which was itself misunderstood) in March of 2020). I proved that not only did we reach herd immunity on that date, we reached this major milestone without anyone being fully vaccinated (two doses plus 3 weeks) which was very important because it showed we didn't need the vaccine at all despite the M.D.T V. Mafia saying we needed 60 – 70%, then 90%, then 98% (Biden) vaccinated before we could reach herd immunity. Remember that?

The public was tricked into thinking they had to get the vaccine to help us reach herd immunity when the truth was, we didn't need even a single person vaccinated. This was incredibly important as was my proof that the vaccine could not block transmission of the virus from person to person. I proved them both over the two-day span of January 14 and January 15, 2021.

I made videos about both of these proofs but no one acknowledged my proofs or even responded. Of course, YouTube was on to me by then and took them down in less than an hour. If the scientific community had acknowledged these two major insights and appreciated their consequences, and had helped get the word out to the public, I believe they (the public) would have rejected the vaccines since they offered almost no benefits and were loaded with risks. The fiasco would have been over as soon as Delta fizzled later in the year. The rise of Omicron was a result of antigenic imprinting brought on by giving vaccines that do not prevent spread during an active pandemic. Omicron was actually a failed variant until the vaccines induced antigenic imprinting.

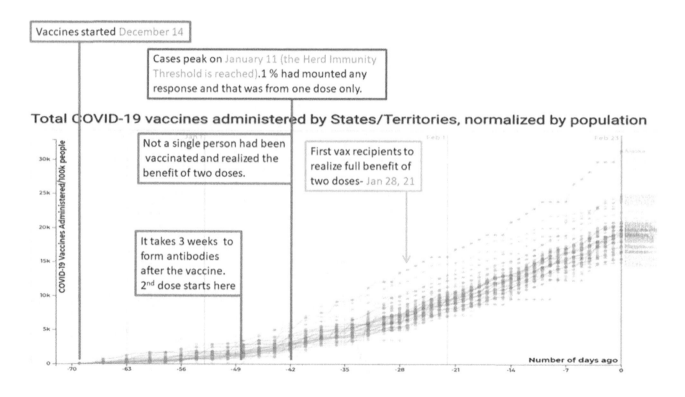

174

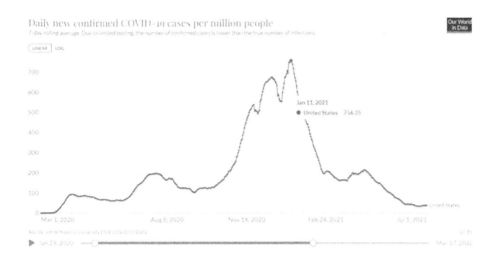

11. Variants of the virus appear & are of great concern.

I believe the purpose of this fiction was to extend the apparent duration of the pandemic & fear for as long as the perpetrators wished it.

While there is controversy on this point, with some physicians believing re-infection by variants to be a serious problem, I think untrustworthy testing and other viruses entirely is the parsimonious explanation.

I come at it as an immunologist. From that vantage point, there is very strong precedent indicating that recovery after infection affords immunity which extends beyond the sequence of the variant which infected the patient, to all variants of SARS-CoV-2.

The number of confirmed re-infections is so small that they are not an issue, epidemiologically speaking.

We have good evidence from those infected by SARS in 2003: they not only have strong T-cell immunity to SARS, but cross-immunity to SARS-CoV-2. This is very important because SARS-CoV-2 is arguably a variant of SARS, being around 20% difference at the sequence level.

Consider this: if our immune systems are able to recognise SARS-CoV-2 as foreign and mount an immune response to it, despite never having seen it before, because of prior immunity conferred by infection years ago by a virus which is 20% different, its logical that variants of SARS-CoV-2, like delta and omicron, will not evade our immunity.

No variant of SARS-CoV-2 differs from the original, Wuhan sequence by more than 3%, and probably less.

Normal rules of immunology apply here. Despite the publicity to the contrary, SARS-CoV-2 mutates relatively slowly and no variant is even close to evading immunity acquired by natural infection.

This is because the human immune system recognises 20-30 different structural motifs in the virus, yet requires only a handful to recall and effective immune memory.

https://www.biorxiv.org/content/10.1101/2020.12.08.416750v1

https://www.biorxiv.org/content/10.1101/2021.02.27.433180v1

The variants story fails to note "Muller's Ratchet", the phenomenon in which variants of a virus, formed in an infected person during viral replication (in which "typographical errors" are made & not corrected) trend to greater transmissibility but lesser lethality. If this was not the case, at some point in human evolution, we would have expected a respiratory viral pandemic to have killed off a substantial proportion of humanity. There is no historical record for such an event.

I do not rule out the possibility that the so-called vaccines are so badly designed that they prevent the establishment of immune memory. If that is true, then the vaccines are worse than failures and it might be possible to be repeatedly infected. This would be a form of acquired immune deficiency.

12.   The only way to end the pandemic is universal vaccination.

This I believe was always the objective of the largely faked pandemic. It's NEVER been the way prior pandemics have ended and there was nothing about this one which should have led us to adopt the extreme risks which were taken & which has resulted in hundreds of thousands, probably millions, of wholly avoidable deaths.   The interventions imposed on the population didn't prevent spread of the virus. Only individual isolation for an open-ended period could do that and that's clearly impossible (hospital patients and residents of care homes have to be cared for at very least and additionally, the nation has to be supplied with food and medicines).

The interventions were useless and hugely burdensome.

Yet we have reached the end of the pandemic, more or less. We would done so faster & with less suffering and death had we adopted measures along the lines proposed in the Great Barrington Declaration and the use of pharmaceutical treatments as they were discovered, plus general improvements to public health, such as encouraging vitamin supplements.

It was NEVER appropriate to attempt to "end the pandemic" with a novel technology vaccine. In a public health mass intervention, safety is the top priority, more so even than effectiveness, because so many people will receive it.

It's simply not possible to obtain data demonstrating adequate longitudinal safety in the time period any pandemic can last.

Those who pushed this line of argument and enabled the gene-based agents to be injected needlessly into billions of innocent people are guilty of crimes against humanity.

It quickly became apparent that natural immunity was stronger than any protection from vaccination and most people were not at risk of severe outcomes if infected.

https://www.medrxiv.org/content/10.1101/2021.08.24.21262415v1

https://brownstone.org/articles/79-research-studies-affirm-naturally-acquired-immunity-to-covid-19-documented-linked-and-quoted/

Even children who were immunocompromised are not at elevated risk from covid-19, so advice that such children should be vaccinated is lethally flawed.

https://pubmed.ncbi.nlm.nih.gov/34785268/

These agents are clearly underperforming against expectations. https://brownstone.org/articles/16-studies-on-vaccine-efficacy/

13.   The new vaccines are safe and effective.

I feel particularly strongly about this claim.

Both components are lies.

I outline the inevitability of the toxicity of all four gene-based agents to the right. Separately, the clinical trials were wholly inadequate. They were conducted in people not most in need of protection from safe & effective vaccines. They were far too short in duration. The endpoints only captured "infection" as measured by an inadequate PCR test and should have been augmented by Sanger sequencing to confirm real infection. Trials were underpowered to detect important endpoints like hospitalisation and death.

There's evidence of fraud in at least one of the pivotal clinical trials. I think there is also clear evidence of manufacturing fraud and regulatory collusion. They should never have been granted EUAs.

The design of the agents called vaccines is very bothersome. Gene-based agents are new in a public health application. Had I been in a regulatory role, I would have informed all the leading R&D companies that I would not approve these without extensive longitudinal studies, meaning they could not receive EUA before early 2022 at the earliest. I would have outright denied their use in children, in pregnancy and in the infected / recovered. Point blank. I'd need years of safe use before contemplating an alteration of this stance.

The basic rules of this new activity, gene-based component vaccines, are (1) to select part of the virus that have no inherent biological action. That rules out spike protein, which we inferred would be very toxic, before they'd even started clinical trials.
https://www.medrxiv.org/content/10.1101/2021.03.05.21252960v1.full
(2) select the genetically most-stable parts of the virus, so we could ignore the gross misrepresentations of variants so slight in difference from the original that we were being toyed with via propaganda. Again, rules out spike protein. (3) choose parts of the virus which are most-different from any human proteins. Once more, spike protein is immediately deselected, otherwise unnecessary risks of autoimmunity are carried forward.

That all four leading actors chose spike protein, against any reasonable selection criteria, leads me to suspect both collusion and malign intent.
Finally, let nature guide us. Against which components of the virus does natural immunity aim? We find 90% of the immune repertoire targets NON-spike protein responses. I rest my case.
https://www.cell.com/immunity/fulltext/S1074-7613(20)30447-7?dgcid=raven_jbs_aip_email
These agents were always going to be toxic. The only question was to what degree? Having selected spike protein to be expressed, a protein which causes blood clotting to be initiated, a risk of thromboembolic adverse events was burned into the design.
Nothing at all limits the amount of spike protein to be made in response to a given dose. Some individuals make a little and only briefly. The other end of a normal range results in synthesis of copious amounts of spike protein for a prolonged period. The locations in which this pathological event occurred, as well as where on the spectrum, in my view played a pivotal role in whether the victim experienced adverse events including death.
There are many other pathologies flowing from the design of these agents, including for the mRNA "vaccines" that lipid nanoparticle formulations leave the injection site and home to liver and ovaries (see footnote 1), among other organs, but this evidence is enough to get started.
https://www.docdroid.net/xq0Z8B0/pfizer-report-japanese-government-pdf#page=15

See here for evidence of clinical trial and other fraud, publicised by Ed Dowd, a former Blackrock investment analyst:

https://www.onenewspage.com/video/20220204/14277521/Edward-Dowd-Interview-portion-on-Steve-Bannons-War.htm

See here for evidence of official data fraud (UK Office of National Statistics): esp 2min 45sec for the heart of the matter.
https://www.bitchute.com/video/KApFxhjiWLqI/

See here for evidence of manufacturing fraud. The same methodology was used to obtain regulatory authorisations and so it is my contention that there is also regulatory fraud.
https://www.bitchute.com/video/4HllyBmOEJeY/

In the Pfizer clinical trial briefing document to FDA which was used for issuing the EUA, on p.40 or thereabout there is a paragraph stating that there were ~2,000 "suspected unconfirmed covid cases". Meaning people were sick with symptoms, but were not tested (otherwise it would be stated that the tests were negative). Of these, in the first 7 days after injection there were 400 in the vaccine arm and 200 in placebo. These subjects were excluded from the dataset used to assess efficacy. It's as clear evidence of fraud as you can get, they admit to it in FDA briefing! Nobody paid any attention to this that I am aware of.
There's also evidence of data fraud in that clinical trial as summarised by Dr Peter Doshi, the deputy editor of the British Medical Journal.

Though many people refuse to accept or even look at the evidence, it is clear that the number of adverse events and deaths soon after c19 vaccination is astonishing and far in excess, in 2021 alone, than all adverse effects and deaths reported to VAERS in the previous 30 years. Here is a simplified view from VAERS.
https://openvaers.com/covid-data/mortality

This excellent presentation by a forensic statistician, well used to presenting analyses for court purposes, dismantles the claims that the vaccines are effective and shows how toxicity is hidden:
https://rumble.com/vtxi1h-open-science-sessions-how-flawed-data-has-driven-the-narrative.html   (see the second half of the recording).

Another paper from the same group, questioning vaccine efficacy:
https://www.researchgate.net/publication/356756711_Latest_statistics_on_England_mortality_data_suggest_systematic_mis-categorisation_of_vaccine_status_and_uncertain_effectiveness_of_Covid-19_vaccination

- Dr. Mike Yeadon

Where Do We Go From Here?

I will explain the etiology of all of this and much more in great detail in my next book, "If Only They Had Listened: *How I Cracked the Biggest Crime in Medical History*" (with the word "Medical" crossed out but you can still read it). Incidentally, all of the insights I'm describing here and elsewhere in the book you are reading now will be proved with a detailed explanation in the coming book which will be available in December, I hope. It's becoming my grand opus. I'm already 250 pages into it and I haven't even scratched the surface. I incorporate the physics that aided me in making all of these insights before anyone else- the "firsts"- and a few that still haven't been recognized by the scientific community- the "onlys"- molecular genetics, immunology, virology and statistical analysis I used over the last two years to make more than 22 of those "firsts" and "onlys" on issues of major importance.

For example, If the public had been able to see my derivation on March 8, 2020 that the IFR was the same as the flu and my demonstrations why lockdowns could not work, they would not have agreed to them and we would have avoided the 150 million deaths that will result from collateral damage associated with those lockdowns; from starvation secondary to supply chain disruptions and from cancer secondary to moratoria placed on all but emergency surgery.

In addition to these two, about half of cancer patients stopped getting chemotherapy, about one third missed routine cancer screening procedures such as colonoscopy, and about one third of children missed their beneficial childhood vaccines.

 In addition to those deaths, If the public had been able to see my proofs that we reached herd immunity without a single person fully-vaccinated on January 11, 2021 along with my proof that the vaccines could not block transmission only four days later, both less than a month after the rollout started, they would have rejected the vaccines and the pandemic would be a distant memory now. We would have avoided the God knows how many deaths we will get from the disease AND the number we have gotten and will get from the vaccine. If we hadn't done the lockdowns and we hadn't done the vaccines, there would have been the same number of deaths as a typical above average flu season- less than the 2017-2018 flu season in fact, when we lost 79,400 people. Remember, the death toll that crossed the million person mark in late May of 2022 was a figure that included deaths "with" and "from" COVID. I think I can prove the actual number in the U.S. was around 150,000 at that time. That was right at two-and-a half seasons of the pandemic so, taking the upper limit, the number of deaths per year was about 60,000; roughly 20,000 lower than the 2017-2018 flu season when there was no mass-testing of asymptomatic people, no school closures, no lockdowns, no ridiculous subsidies to big business and hospitals, and no one lost their job. Oh, and I forgot- the 7+ trillion dollars we wasted on this man-made disaster.

Considering that there were no flu deaths in the entire world in 2020- I never could figure out how this could be possible (unless the flu deaths were assigned to COVID or entire virus populations really do get displaced by the dominant one of the moment, the sum of COVID deaths + flu deaths was right at the upper limit of what it always is- around 60,000 deaths that year. There is a lot of speculation here but it is based on the hard numbers from Sweden as per slide #7 in the "9 Most Important Slides of the Pandemic. Yes, ladies and gentlemen you have been taken, and are still being taken, for a horrible ride with the inflation and recession this fraud will likely cause. More mask mandates are being threatened now- Dr. Fauci did so just this morning- and the graphs of cases vs. time look very, very bad with higher lows and what is nearing higher highs. The people who perpetrated this evil on our innocent fellow citizens are the Villains listed in this book. There are a others who slipped under my radar. I'll get them in the next edition if there needs to be one.

Recently, I heard Drs. Fauci, Collins, Birx and several others trying to rewrite history to mitigate their culpability in the death and destruction they wrought, trying to make us overlook what was done by talking about having to "learn from the mistakes that were made this time so we can be ready for the next pandemic".

I SAY NO! We shouldn't be talking about what we're going to change for the next pandemic until we fully prosecute every one of these criminals for what they did during COVID-19. We need to set up Nuremberg-type hearings as soon as possible and put those found guilty of all these murders in prison for life. The Nuremberg Trials were brought to order, in part, to heal the world after World War II. We need to heal these wounds. The only way we are going to do that is by seeing those responsible for the murder and mayhem, prosecuted according to the law.

The wounds I speak of will get deeper and more painful, sadly, as more and more of the public comes to understand my proofs that there was planning at the highest level, malfeasance and collusion between the vaccine-makers, that the SARS-2 virus was synthesized in a lab, etc. So ask for evidence from anyone who says this is still unknown- that there is a possibility SARS-2 arose from natural zoonotic spillover from a bat or intermediate host. And ask for evidence from anyone who tries to tell you the vaccine trials were run properly. The vaccine trials for adults and children were riddled with fraud and deceit by our own FDA whose mission it is, to protect the citizens of the United States of America from unsafe food and drugs. It is almost inconceivable but the FDA, CDC, NIH and NIAID have become corrupted so profoundly by the influences of the pharmaceutical industry as to approve these experimental formulations without adequate justification, putting the lives of six-month-old babies at risk for a negative benefit. That's right. It is now crystal clear and has been so for months. At almost any age, or perhaps all ages, people would have been better off *not* getting the vaccines. It appears there was some benefit against COVID-19- but how can you believe any of their figures after they've lied about so much of it?

It does us no good to say something like, "The FDA is in the pocket of Big Pharma. That's why they engaged in poor practices like visiting only one out of 99 Moderna trial injection sites and authorized the Pfizer vaccines for emergency use in small children when there was no justification for it." Focus must be placed on *individual committee members* who voted to approve when there was no scientific justification for it. Individual people who must be called out and punished severely for the lives they destroyed and lost and for the lives that will be destroyed and lost in the future. This book listed the names. Ask them for an explanation. It is unconscionable what was done. People keep talking about the "mistakes" that were made this time. These weren't "mistakes". This was deliberate. It was planned. I'd stake my life on it. We are not going to let these criminals get away with this by sweeping it under the   "Let bygones be bygones, we'll do better next time", rug.

Who is "WE"? It is you. It is me. There is no one else.

Acknowledgements

Many people have been instrumental in the writing of this book.

Many thanks go to: George Todd, who helped me with last minute editing, Laura Crawford, who helped educate me on the situation in Australia and New Zealand, Rhonda Hutchinson and Pascal Plamondon who did the same for Canada, David Tohir who sent me many informative articles over the last two years and set me up in the F.R.O.G. to write the final chapters Thanks also to Dr. Carmen Martinez who lent me a room to write when I was in a jam and Sarai Williams who helped with formatting.

Thank you so much to the wonderful employees of Panara Bread on A1A in Ponte Vedra, Florida for letting me write all night in their outside café for a week when my WiFi went down. Finally, once again, many, many thanks to Dr. Mike Yeadon who went above and beyond the call of duty in answering my request to contribute his expertise to this book. I asked him for a list, he sent me a chapter.

Note: I have no suicidal tendencies whatsoever

APPENDICES

APPENDIX I

YouTube's Covid-19 Medical Misinformation Policy followed by their Vaccine Misinformation Policy

COVID-19 medical misinformation policy

The safety of our creators, viewers, and partners is our highest priority. We look to each of you to help us protect this unique and vibrant community. It's important you understand our Community Guidelines, and the role they play in our shared responsibility to keep YouTube safe. Take the time to carefully read the policy below. You can also check out this page for a full list of our guidelines.

YouTube doesn't allow content about COVID-19 that poses a serious risk of egregious harm.

YouTube doesn't allow content that spreads medical misinformation that contradicts local health authorities' (LHA) or the World Health Organization's (WHO) medical information about COVID-19. This is limited to content that contradicts WHO or local health authorities' guidance on:

Treatment
Prevention
Diagnosis
Transmission
The existence of COVID-19

Note: YouTube's policies on COVID-19 are subject to change in response to changes to global or local health authorities' guidance on the virus. There may be a delay between new LHA/WHO guidance and policy updates given the frequency with which this guidance changes, and our policies may not cover all LHA/WHO guidance related to COVID-19.

Our COVID-19 policies were first published on May 20, 2020.

What this policy means for you
If you're posting content
Don't post content on YouTube if it includes any of the following:

Treatment misinformation:

Content that encourages the use of home remedies, prayer, or rituals in place of medical treatment such as consulting a doctor or going to the hospital

Content that claims that there's a guaranteed cure for COVID-19

Content that recommends use of Ivermectin or Hydroxychloroquine for the treatment of COVID-19

Claims that Hydroxychloroquine is an effective treatment for COVID-19

Categorical claims that Ivermectin is an effective treatment for COVID-19

Claims that Ivermectin and Hydroxychloroquine are safe to use in the prevention of COVID-19

Other content that discourages people from consulting a medical professional or seeking medical advice

Prevention misinformation: Content that promotes prevention methods that contradict local health authorities or WHO.

Claims that there is a guaranteed prevention method for COVID-19

Claims that any medication or vaccination is a guaranteed prevention method for COVID-19

Content that recommends use of Ivermectin or Hydroxychloroquine for the prevention of COVID-19

Claims that Ivermectin and Hydroxychloroquine are safe to use in the prevention of COVID-19

Claims about COVID-19 vaccinations that contradict expert consensus from local health authorities or WHO

Claims that an approved COVID-19 vaccine will cause death, infertility, miscarriage, autism, or contraction of other infectious diseases

Claims that an approved COVID-19 vaccine will contain substances that are not on the vaccine ingredient list, such as biological matter from fetuses (e.g. fetal tissue, fetal cell lines) or animal products

Claims that an approved COVID-19 vaccine will contain substances or devices meant to track or identify those who've received it

Claims that COVID-19 vaccines will make people who receive them magnetic

Claims that an approved COVID-19 vaccine will alter a person's genetic makeup

Claims that COVID-19 vaccines do not reduce risk of serious illness or death

Claims that any vaccine causes contraction of COVID-19

Claims that a specific population will be required (by any entity except for a government) to take part in vaccine trials or receive the vaccine first

Content that promotes the use of unapproved or homemade COVID-19 vaccines

Instructions to counterfeit vaccine certificates, or offers of sale for such documents

Diagnostic misinformation: Content that promotes diagnostic information that contradicts local health authorities or WHO.

Claims that approved COVID-19 tests are dangerous or cause negative physical health effects

Claims that approved COVID-19 tests cannot diagnose COVID-19

Transmission misinformation: Content that promotes transmission information that contradicts local health authorities or WHO.

Content that claims that COVID-19 is not caused by a viral infection

Content that claims COVID-19 is not contagious

Content that claims that COVID-19 cannot spread in certain climates or geographies

Content that claims that any group or individual has immunity to the virus or cannot transmit the virus

Content that denies the existence of COVID-19:

Denial that COVID-19 exists
Claims that people have not died or gotten sick from COVID-19
Claims that the death rate of COVID-19 is equal to or less than that of the common cold or seasonal flu
Claims that COVID-19 is equal to or less transmissible than the common cold or seasonal flu
Claims that the symptoms of COVID-19 are never severe
This policy applies to videos, video descriptions, comments, live streams, and any other YouTube product or feature. Keep in mind that this isn't a complete list. Please note these policies also apply to external links in your content. This can include clickable URLs, verbally directing users to other sites in video, as well as other forms.

Examples
Here are some examples of content that's not allowed on YouTube:

Denial that COVID-19 exists
Claims that people have not died from COVID-19
Claims that any vaccine is a guaranteed prevention method for COVID-19
Claims that a specific treatment or medicine is a guaranteed cure for COVID-19
Claims that hydroxychloroquine saves people from COVID-19
Promotion of MMS (Miracle Mineral Solution) for the treatment of COVID-19
Claims that certain people have immunity to COVID-19 due to their race or nationality
Encouraging taking home remedies instead of getting medical treatment when sick
Discouraging people from consulting a medical professional if they're sick
Content that claims that holding your breath can be used as a diagnostic test for COVID-19
Videos alleging that if you avoid Asian food, you won't get the coronavirus
Videos alleging that setting off fireworks can clean the air of the virus and will prevent the spread of the virus
Claims that COVID-19 is caused by radiation from 5G networks
Videos alleging that the COVID-19 test is the cause of the virus
Claims that countries with hot climates will not experience the spread of the virus
Claims that COVID-19 vaccines kill people who receive them
Claims that COVID-19 vaccines are a means of population reduction
Videos claiming that COVID-19 vaccines contain fetal tissue
Claims that the flu vaccine causes contraction of COVID-19
Claims that the flu is more contagious than COVID-19
Claims that COVID-19 vaccines cause contraction of other infectious diseases or makes people more vulnerable to contraction of other infectious diseases
Claims that COVID-19 vaccines contain a microchip or tracking device
Claims that achieving herd immunity through natural infection is safer than vaccinating the population
Claims that COVID-19 never causes serious symptoms or hospitalization
Claims that the death rate from the seasonal flu is higher than the death rate of COVID-19
Claims that people are immune to the virus based on their race
Claims that children cannot or do not contract COVID-19

Claims that there have not been cases or deaths in countries where cases or deaths have been confirmed by local health authorities or the WHO

Educational, documentary, scientific or artistic content

We may allow content that violates the misinformation policies noted on this page if that content includes additional context in the video, audio, title, or description. This is not a pass to promote misinformation. Additional context may include countervailing views from local health authorities or medical experts. We may also make exceptions if the purpose of the content is to condemn, dispute, or satirize misinformation that violates our policies. We may also make exceptions for content showing an open public forum, like a protest or public hearing, provided the content does not aim to promote misinformation that violates our policies.

What happens if content violates this policy

If your content violates this policy, we'll remove the content and send you an email to let you know. If this is your first time violating our Community Guidelines, you'll likely get a warning with no penalty to your channel. If it's not, we may issue a strike against your channel. If you get 3 strikes within 90 days, your channel will be terminated. You can learn more about our strikes system here.

We may terminate your channel or account for repeated violations of the Community Guidelines or Terms of Service. We may also terminate your channel or account after a single case of severe abuse, or when the channel is dedicated to a policy violation. You can learn more about channel or account terminations here.

Vaccine misinformation policy

YouTube doesn't allow content that poses a serious risk of egregious harm by spreading medical misinformation about currently administered vaccines that are approved and confirmed to be safe and effective by local health authorities and by the World Health Organization (WHO). This is limited to content that contradicts local health authorities' or the WHO's guidance on vaccine safety, efficacy, and ingredients.

What this policy means for you

If you're posting content

Don't post content on YouTube if it includes harmful misinformation about currently approved and administered vaccines on any of the following:

Vaccine safety: content alleging that vaccines cause chronic side effects, outside of rare side effects that are recognized by health authorities

Efficacy of vaccines: content claiming that vaccines do not reduce transmission or contraction of disease

Ingredients in vaccines: content misrepresenting the substances contained in vaccines

This policy applies to videos, video descriptions, comments, live streams, and any other YouTube product or feature. Keep in mind that this isn't a complete list. Please note these policies also apply to external links in your content. This can include clickable URLs, verbally directing users to other sites in video, as well as other forms.

Examples
Here are some examples of content that's not allowed on YouTube:

Claims that vaccines cause chronic side effects such as:
Cancer
Diabetes
Other chronic side effects
Claims that vaccines do not reduce risk of contracting illness
Claims that vaccines contain substances that are not on the vaccine ingredient list, such as biological matter from fetuses (e.g. fetal tissue, fetal cell lines) or animal byproducts
Claims that vaccines contain substances or devices meant to track or identify those who've received them
Claims that vaccines alter a person's genetic makeup
Claims that the MMR vaccine causes autism
Claims that vaccines are part of a depopulation agenda
Claims that the flu vaccine causes chronic side effects such as infertility
Claims that the HPV vaccine causes chronic side effects such as paralysis
Educational, scientific, artistic, or testimonial content
YouTube may allow content that violates the misinformation policies noted on this page if that content includes additional context in the video, audio, title, or description. This is not a pass to promote misinformation. Additional context may include countervailing views from local health authorities or medical experts. We may also make exceptions if the purpose of the content is to condemn, dispute, or satirize misinformation that violates our policies. We may also make exceptions for content showing an open public forum, like a protest or public hearing, provided the content does not aim to promote misinformation that violates our policies.

YouTube also believes people should be able to share their own experiences, including personal experiences with vaccinations. This means we may make exceptions for content in which creators describe firsthand experiences from themselves or their family. At the same time, we recognize there is a difference between sharing personal experiences and promoting misinformation about vaccines. To address this balance, we will still remove content or channels if they include other policy violations or demonstrate a pattern of promoting vaccine misinformation.

What happens if content violates this policy
If your content violates this policy, we'll remove the content and send you an email to let you know. If this is your first time violating our Community Guidelines, you'll likely get a warning with no penalty to your channel. If it's not, we may issue a strike against your channel. If you get 3 strikes within 90 days, your channel will be terminated. You can learn more about our strikes system here.

We may terminate your channel or account for repeated violations of the Community Guidelines or Terms of Service. We may also terminate your channel or account after a single case of severe abuse, or when the channel is dedicated to a policy violation. You can learn more about channel or account terminations here.

APPENDIX II

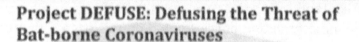

PROPOSAL: VOLUME I
DARPA – PREEMPT (HR001118S0017)
LEAD ORGANIZATION: EcoHealth Alliance (Other Nonprofit)
OTHER TEAM MEMBERS:
Duke NUS Medical School (Other Educational)
University of North Carolina (Other Educational)
Wuhan Institute of Virology (Other Educational)
USGS National Wildlife Health Center (Other Nonprofit)
Palo Alto Research Center (Large Business)

Project DEFUSE: Defusing the Threat of Bat-borne Coronaviruses

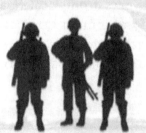

Principal Investigator and Technical Point of Contact	Administrative Point of Contact
Peter Daszak, Ph.D.	Luke Hamel
EcoHealth Alliance	EcoHealth Alliance
460 West 34th Street, 17th Floor	460 West 34th Street, 17th Floor
New York, NY 10001	New York, NY 10001
(p) 212-380-4474	(p) 646-868-4709
(e) daszak@ecohealthalliance.org	(e) hamel@ecohealthalliance.org
(f) 212-380-4465	(f) 212-380-4465

Identifying Number: HR001118S0017-PREEMPT-PA-001
Award Instrument Requested: Grant
Places and Periods of Performance: 12/1/18 - 5/31/22; Palo Alto, CA; Kunming and Wuhan, China; Chapel Hill, NC; New York, NY; Singapore; Madison, WI
Total funds requested: $14,209,245

Section II   A. EXECUTIVE SUMMARY

<u>Technical Approach:</u> Our goal is to defuse the potential for spillover of novel bat-origin high-zoonotic risk SARS-related coronaviruses in Asia. **In TA1** we will intensively sample bats at our field sites where we have identified high spillover risk SARSr-CoVs. We will sequence their spike proteins, reverse engineer them to conduct binding assays, and insert them into bat SARSr-CoV (WIV1, SHC014) backbones (these use bat-SARSr-CoV backbones, not SARS-CoV, and are exempt from dual-use and gain of function concerns) to infect humanized mice and assess capacity to cause SARS-like disease. Our modeling team will use these data to build **machine-learning genotype-phenotype models** of viral evolution and spillover risk. We will uniquely validate these with serology from previously-collected human samples via LIPS assays that assess which spike proteins allow spillover into people. We will build **host-pathogen spatial models** to predict the bat species composition of caves across Southeast Asia, parameterized with a full inventory of host-virus distribution at our field test sites, three caves in Yunnan Province, China, and a series of unique global datasets on bat host-viral relationships. By the end of Y1, we will create a prototype app for the warfighter that identifies the likelihood of bats harboring dangerous viral pathogens at any site across Asia.

In **TA2**, we will evaluate two approaches to reduce SARSr-CoV shedding in cave bats: (1) **Broadscale immune boosting**, in which we will inoculate bats with immune modulators to upregulate their innate immune response and downregulate viral replication; **(2) Targeted immune boosting**, in which we will inoculate bats with novel chimeric polyvalent recombinant spike proteins plus the immune modulator to enhance innate immunity against specific, high-risk viruses. We will trial inoculum delivery methods on captive bats including a novel automated aerosolization system, transdermal nanoparticle application and edible adhesive gels. We will use stochastic simulation modeling informed by field and experimental data to characterize viral dynamics in our cave test sites, maximize timing, inoculation protocol, delivery method and efficacy of viral suppression. The most effective biologicals will be trialed in our test cave sites in Yunnan Province, with reduction in viral shedding as proof-of-concept.

<u>Management Approach:</u> Members of our collaborative group have worked together on bats and their viruses for over 15 years. The lead organization, EcoHealth Alliance, will oversee all work. EHA staff will develop models to evaluate the probability of specific SARS-related CoV spillover, and identify the most effective strategy for delivery of both immune boosting and immune targeting inocula. Specific work will be subcontracted to the following organizations:

- Prof. Baric, Univ. N. Carolina, will lead targeted immune boosting work, building on his two-decade track record of reverse-engineering CoV and other virus spike proteins.
- Prof. Wang, Duke-Natl. Univ. Singapore, will lead work on broadscale immune boosting, building on his group's pioneering work on bat immunity.
- Dr. Shi, Wuhan Institute of Virology will conduct viral testing on all collected samples, binding assays and some humanized mouse work.
- Dr. Rocke, USGS National Wildlife Health Center will optimize delivery of immune modulating biologicals, building on her vaccine delivery work in wildlife, including bats.
- Dr. Unidad, Palo Alto Research Center will lead development of novel delivery automated aerosolization mechanism for immune boosting molecules.

We are requesting $14,209,245 total funds for this project across 3.5 project years.

To characterize spillover risk of SARSr-CoV quasispecies (QS), the Wuhan Institute of Virology team (WIV) will test bat fecal, oral, and blood samples for SARSr-CoVs by PCR. We will collect viral load data from fresh fecal pellets. SARSr-CoV spike proteins will be sequenced, viral recombination events identified, and isolates used to identify strains that can replicate in human cells. The Univ. N. Carolina (UNC) team will reverse-engineer spike proteins of a large sample of high- and low-risk viruses for further characterization. This will effectively freeze the QS we analyze at t=0. These QS_0 strain viral spike glycoproteins will be synthesized, and those binding to human cell receptor ACE2 will be inserted into SARSr-CoV backbones (non-DURC, non-GoF), and inoculated into humanized mice to assess capacity to cause SARS-like disease, efficacy of monoclonal therapies, the inhibitor GS-5734[8] or vaccines against SARS-CoV[8-12].

Prof. Baric (UNC) will lead the targeted immune boosting work. We will develop recombinant chimeric spike-proteins[22] from known SARSr-CoVs, and those characterized by DEFUSE. Using details of SARS S protein structure and host cell binding[23] we will sequence, reconstruct and characterize spike trimers and receptor binding domains of SARSr-CoVs, incorporate them into nanoparticles or raccoon poxvirus-vectors for delivery to bats[10,24-27]. In combination with immune-boosting small molecules, we will use these to boost immune memory in adult bats previously exposed to SARSr-CoVs, taking the best candidate forward for field-testing. Recombinant S glycoprotein-based constructs with immunogenic blocks from across group 2B SARSr-CoVs should induce broadscale adaptive immune responses that reduce heterogeneous virus burdens in bats and transmission risk to people[28,29]. Innate immune damping is highly conserved in all bat species tested so far. We will use the unique Duke-NUS

INDEX

189

Made in the USA
Las Vegas, NV
07 December 2022

61393473R00116